Other monographs in the series, *Major Problems in Clinical Pediatrics*:

Avery: *The Lung and Its Disorders in the Newborn Infant*—published in April, 1964.

Cornblath and Schwartz: *Disorders of Carbohydrate Metabolism in Infancy*—to be published early in 1966.

Oski and Naiman: *Hematologic Problems of the Newborn*—to be published in 1966.

Rowe and Mehrizi: *The Neonate with Congenital Heart Disease*—to be published in 1966.

RHEUMATIC FEVER
Diagnosis, Management and Prevention

By

Milton Markowitz, A.B., M.D.

Assistant Pediatrician-in-Chief, Sinai
Hospital of Baltimore; Associate Professor
of Pediatrics, Johns Hopkins University School
of Medicine; Pediatrician-in-Charge, Rheumatic
Fever Clinic, Harriet Lane Home Service,
Children's Medical and Surgical Center,
The Johns Hopkins Hospital

and

Ann Gayler Kuttner, B.S., Ph.D., M.D.

Associate Professor of Pediatrics, Emeritus, New
York University, Bellevue Medical Center;
Visiting Scientist, Streptococcal Disease
Laboratory, Sinai Hospital of Baltimore

*With a special chapter on
Community Health Services by*

Leon Gordis, A.B., M.D.

Field Officer, Heart Disease Control
Program, U.S. Public Health Service; Fellow
in Pediatrics, Sinai Hospital and The
Johns Hopkins Hospital

Volume II in the Series
**MAJOR PROBLEMS IN
CLINICAL PEDIATRICS**

ALEXANDER J. SCHAFFER
Consulting Editor

W. B. Saunders Company, Philadelphia and London

Reprinted September, 1965

Rheumatic Fever

Affectionately Dedicated
to
SELMA L. MARKOWITZ AND REBECCA C. LANCEFIELD

Preface

In 1888, Cheadle, in a series of lectures on rheumatic fever commented: "There is perhaps no serious disease more familiar to us than acute articular rheumatism; it is one of the disorders most commonly seen in the wards of a general hospital; it is constantly encountered in private practice. . . ."

Forty years later, Glover (1930) noted that "the incidence of acute rheumatism seems to show that it, like tuberculosis, is slowly but surely being conquered. . . . We seem to be seeing the same process of epidemiologic obsolescence in acute rheumatism that Creighton saw in smallpox. . . . But whilst we appreciate this cheering decline in the incidence of rheumatic fever, we are still painfully aware of the high incidence in children of the major and minor stigmata of the acute rheumatic infection, and of those many patients who, in what should be their happy youth or vigorous manhood, perish slowly of rheumatic heart disease.

"The triumph over acute rheumatism, of which this decline is but the herald, is yet far off. It must but spur us on to further effort, first to prevent as far as possible the infection of children, secondly to supervise those who may have been infected, thirdly to provide institutional treatment for those seriously infected to insure them the fairest chance of recovering from their carditis without permanent damage to the heart."

The progress made during the interim between Cheadle and Glover was directly related to the decline in poverty, malnutrition, overcrowding, and substandard housing. What advances have been made since 1930? Social conditions have continued to improve. The relationship of group A streptococci to rheumatic fever has been firmly established and it has become clear that social factors affect the incidence of rheumatic fever because they are related to streptococcal infections. Antimicrobial agents were developed to combat and prevent streptococcal infections and thus reduce the incidence of initial and recurrent attacks of rheumatic fever.

Rheumatic fever continues to decline and debilitating heart disease is less common. But Glover's prediction of obsolescence has as yet not been fulfilled. Why is this so? Important predisposing factors such as poverty and overcrowded slums have not been eliminated. Children with rheumatic fever go unrecognized because there has been no major advance made in our ability to diagnose subacute attacks of this disease. Despite the known relationship of group A streptococci to rheumatic fever, the pathogenesis has not been elucidated and curative therapy is not available. Initial attacks which might possibly be prevented still occur because many children do not receive medical attention for antecedent infections. Furthermore, the diagnosis of streptococcal pharyngitis is either frequently not made or inadequate treatment is prescribed. Recurrent attacks in known rheumatic subjects also still occur because proven prophylactic measures are all too often not carried out consistently.

Thus, rheumatic fever remains a challenge. Its ultimate eradication depends on further improvement in living conditions, better methods to prevent streptococcal infections, and a more complete understanding of the pathogenesis of the disease. However, with the knowledge currently available, physicians can reduce the incidence of severe rheumatic heart disease and by preventing initial attacks eventually make rheumatic fever a truly rare disease.

In this monograph the biology of group A streptococci is briefly reviewed, and the serologic and epidemiologic data that link these organisms with rheumatic fever are summarized. The changing pattern, clinical manifestations, diagnosis, and treatment as well as the regimens effective for the prevention of recurrences and initial attacks are discussed. No attempt has been made to include an exhaustive review of the literature. Knowledge has advanced much more slowly than the number of papers written on the subject would indicate.

The initial stimulus for our work in the field of rheumatic fever was provided by Dr. Alfred E. Cohn and Dr. Homer F. Swift. Over the years the authors have benefited greatly from the advice and counsel of Dr. Rebecca C. Lancefield.

We were first associated in the study of rheumatic fever at Irvington House. Subsequently the interest in rheumatic fever was encouraged by the late Dr. Francis F. Schwentker and by Dr. Harry H. Gordon. In recent years Dr. Robert E. Cooke, Dr. Eugene Kaplan, and Dr. Helen B. Taussig have provided the opportunities for further study of rheumatic fever.

We are grateful to Dr. Leon Sokoloff for helpful suggestions regarding the chapter on pathology. We are especially indebted to Dr. Alexander J. Schaffer for reviewing the entire text. We would also like to express our thanks to Dr. Catherine C. Neill, Dr. Bernard Tabatznik, and Dr. Leon Gordis for reading and criticizing various sections. We gratefully acknowledge the expert secretarial assistance of Mrs. Vida Hall and express our thanks to Mr. Harold Thomas for charts and photographs and to Mrs. Ethel McConahy for checking the bibliography.

Some of the research studies included in this monograph were supported in part by research grant HE-05555 from the National Institutes of Health, Public Health Service, Bethesda, Maryland.

Foreword

We are pleased to be able to present this volume as the second in the series of Major Problems in Clinical Pediatrics. Our pleasure derives in large part from our long association with both authors and from the high places they have attained in our esteem.

Ann Kuttner began her medical life as a bacteriologist, earning a Ph.D. in that subject and serving as bacteriologist at Columbia, and later at the Hospital of the Rockefeller Institute. Here she developed her abiding interest in the streptococcus while working with Homer Smith and Rebecca Lancefield. She then took her M.D. degree at The Johns Hopkins where she simultaneously acted as bacteriologist to the Harriet Lane Home. Since then she has served in several places as physician and bacteriologist, notably in Peiping, in Cooperstown, at Harvard, and at New York University. During two tours of duty at Irvington House as Chief Physician and Director of Research she became an expert in the clinical aspects of Rheumatic Fever and made valuable contributions to knowledge concerning its etiology. We are happy that she is now with us in Baltimore on leave from New York University as a Visiting Scientist at the Sinai Hospital of Baltimore.

She is presently working closely on a research project with the co-author, Milton Markowitz. Dr. Markowitz obtained his M.D. from Syracuse University School of Medicine, interned, served throughout World War II as a medical officer in the U.S. Navy, then spent a year at Irvington House under Dr. Kuttner. His lifelong preoccupation with rheumatic diseases originated then. After completing his residency training at The Johns Hopkins Harriet Lane Home he became my associate in the practice of pediatrics. During the fourteen years of our association he became not only one of the best clinicians I have ever known but he assisted me mightily in my gropings for knowledge concerning the newborn infant. In addition, he still found time to perfect himself in the subspecialties of cardiology and rheumatology, and to carry out researches in these fields. When these burdens became too heavy for one man to carry he left practice to become Assistant Chief of the Department of Pediatrics of the Sinai Hospital of Baltimore and Director of the Subdepartment of Rheumatic Fever and Rheumatoid Arthritis at the Harriet Lane Home.

We cite these *curricula vitae* in detail in order to demonstrate how well qualified this pair is to write the kind of monograph we desired, and which they have indeed written. It examines the questions of pathology, etiology, and pathogenesis in detail, pointing out what is known and what remains to be learned in these areas. It discusses the often knotty problems of diagnosis, differential diagnosis, and treatment with the *expertise* of doctors who have been confronted with these situations many times a week for many years.

We believe Drs. Markowitz and Kuttner have assembled all the worthwhile information on this subject, and have been able to combine this with their own rich funds of experience in a form which renders this monograph immediately useful to the pediatrician and general practitioner who wishes to deal properly with these disorders.

Alexander J. Schaffer

Contents

Chapter Eleven

Chapter Twelve

Chapter Thirteen

Chapter Fourteen

Chapter Fifteen

Appendix 1.

Chapter One

THE CHANGING PATTERN
OF RHEUMATIC FEVER

During the past 40 years the epidemiology of rheumatic fever has undergone striking changes. Rheumatic heart disease is less prevalent among school children and young adults than it was a few decades ago. This decline may be due to changes in either the incidence or severity of rheumatic fever, or in both. In the opinion of most observers in this country and in England, acute rheumatic fever is less common than formerly although there are no accurate data to prove this impression. There is no doubt, however, that the severity of rheumatic fever has diminished. Evidence indicative of these changes and their possible causes are reviewed in this chapter.

INCIDENCE OF ACUTE RHEUMATIC FEVER

Acute rheumatic fever is not a universally reportable disease. Data on incidence* have been compiled, therefore, from various sources, such as morbidity surveys, hospital admissions, case registries, and health department statistics. Data obtained from these sources are generally incomplete and cannot be readily combined because the criteria used for diagnosis are not uniform. In addition, many subclinical cases of rheumatic fever are not recognized until heart disease becomes manifest and such cases are therefore not included in statistics from any of these sources.

* Incidence of acute rheumatic fever is defined as the frequency of its occurrence in a defined population during a stated period of time.

1

Despite these limitations certain trends can be detected from available reports.

Morbidity Surveys

Stamler (1962), using data obtained from the Department of Health Heart Disease Control Program, estimated that the incidence of acute rheumatic fever in Chicago was 50 per 100,000 children aged 5 to 15 years. In a report by Collins (1947) covering six different surveys conducted during an earlier period (1928 to 1943), the attack rate was 100 to 120 per 100,000 children. Collins' studies were carried out in different parts of the country in populations which may have been very different from that of metropolitan Chicago. Nevertheless, the data suggest that a significant decline in the incidence of acute rheumatic fever has occurred over the past 20 to 30 years.

Hospital Admissions

Mayer et al. (1963) reviewed the rheumatic fever admissions to the pediatric service of Bellevue Hospital in New York City for a 24 year period, 1935 to 1958. The total number of admissions decreased from 368 in 1935 to 1942 to 229 in 1951 to 1958. However this decrease was due chiefly to a decline in the incidence of chorea. If "pure" chorea is excluded, the decline was less striking, 263 to 200. Massell and co-workers (1964) studied admissions to a special institution for rheumatic fever (The House of the Good Samaritan) over a 40 year period. The number of admissions decreased significantly only after 1956. A more striking downward trend occurred in the incidence of patients with chorea, similar to that reported by Mayer et al. (1963). Massell et al. (1964) reported that from 1921 to 1925, 43 per cent of the patients admitted had chorea, whereas from 1956 to 1960 only 15 per cent of the admissions showed this manifestation.

The decrease in the number of admissions with acute rheumatic fever, exclusive of those with "pure" chorea, was not marked in the data reported by these two groups of investigators. Hospital admissions, however, are not entirely reliable indicators of the frequency of a disease in the general population, since they may reflect local admission policies and the interest of the medical staff at a particular time. However, the findings observed in both institutions indicate that the incidence of chorea has clearly declined. The reason for this unusual change in the clinical pattern is not known. Severe epistaxis is another clinical feature which has become much less common.

Case Registries

A number of localities have established registries of rheumatic subjects who receive prophylactic medication. In general, data from case registries indicate that there are more patients with rheumatic fever than is generally appreciated. Unfortunately, statistics obtained from case registries are not entirely reliable because it is often not possible to verify the diagnosis. In a study by Robinson (1956) based on the San Francisco case registry, a fourfold decline in the number of initial attacks of rheumatic fever was noted between 1945 and 1955.

Health Department Statistics

Nationwide statistics on incidence of acute rheumatic fever in the United States are particularly inadequate. In 1962, 7306 cases of acute rheumatic fever were recorded in 31 states where the disease is reportable. Since most cases are not reported, however, this number probably represents only a fraction of the total incidence. In a study done in Minnesota, for example, physicians reported an average of 187 cases annually to the Department of Health between 1950 and 1954. A more careful survey based on questionnaires to all physicians in the state indicated that approximately 1800 children under 15 years of age had rheumatic fever in 1955, 10 times the annual figure reported for the previous five years (Rosenfeld, 1958).

PREVALENCE OF RHEUMATIC HEART DISEASE

The prevalence* of rheumatic heart disease has been estimated in children chiefly from school surveys, and in young adults from preinduction military examinations and college student surveys.

School Children Surveys

A number of observers have conducted surveys on the prevalence of rheumatic heart disease among school children. It must be emphasized that unless the children with suspected heart disease are carefully screened, the data obtained cannot be considered meaningful. For example, in one study of 4599 school children with suspected heart disease, 85 per cent were found to have no evidence of heart disease on further examination (Friedman and Wells, 1956).

The studies listed in Table 1 were carried out in individuals of comparable ages from cities in the northern temperate zone. All suspected cases were re-examined. The prevalence of rheumatic heart disease in studies done between 1920 and 1934 ranged between 4.3 and 5.0 per 1000 school children. The surveys conducted between 1948 and 1960

* Prevalence is defined as the number of patients with rheumatic heart disease at any one time in a given population group.

Table 1. Prevalence of Rheumatic Heart Disease among School
Children: Results of Selected Surveys

Location	Date	Age Group	Rate per 1000	Reference
New York City	1920	6-17	4.3	Halsey (1921)
Boston	1926	6-17	4.5	Robey (1927)
Philadelphia	1934	6-18	5.0	Cahan (1937)
Toronto	1948-1949	5-15	1.6	Gardiner and Keith (1951)
Buffalo	1949-1952	5-18	1.8	Mattison et al. (1953)
Chicago	1959-1960	6-13	1.3	Miller et al. (1962)
New York City	1961	5-18	1.6	Brownell and Stix (1963)

showed a rate of 1.3 to 1.8 per 1000. These data indicate that the prevalence of rheumatic heart disease among children is low at present compared with reports from previous decades. Studies have shown that congenital heart disease may be slightly more common among school children than rheumatic heart disease. Mustacchi et al. (1963) found congenital defects of the heart and great vessels in 2 per 1000 school children in San Francisco. A mass survey among Chicago elementary school children yielded similar results (Miller et al., 1962).

Military Registrants

Rheumatic heart disease was the chief cardiovascular cause for rejection from military service during World War II. Among two million selectees between the ages of 21 and 36, 96,000 were found unfit because of heart disease and of these individuals, approximately 50 per cent suffered from rheumatic heart disease (Fenn et al., 1944). RuDusky (1963) studied the cardiac findings among more than 20,000 men of military age examined in 1960 to 1962. This observer found a prevalence of rheumatic heart disease of 8.8 per 1000, a decrease of 63 per cent from the figure obtained 20 years earlier (Table 2).

Table 2. A Comparison of Per Cent of Patients Rejected from Military
Service for Rheumatic Heart Disease, 1941 to 1943 and 1960 to 1962[*]

	1941-1943	1960-1962
No. Registrants	2,000,000	20,597
% Rejected	2.4	0.88

[*] Modified from RuDusky, B. M.: J.A.M.A. 185:1004, 1963.

College Student Surveys

The U.S. Public Health Service and the American College Health Association have recently completed an extensive study of the prevalence of rheumatic heart disease among college students (Marienfeld et al.,

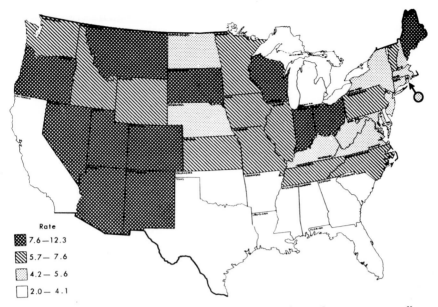

Figure 1. Prevalence rates of current rheumatic heart disease among college freshmen by state of residence. (From Marienfeld et al.: Public Health Rep. 79:789, 1964.)

1964). Freshman students were surveyed during a five year period, 1956 to 1960. Physical examinations of 517,129 individuals revealed a national prevalence rate of rheumatic disease of 5.7 per 1000 students. There was considerable variation among the individual states as is shown in Figure 1. The highest rates were found in the northern temperate zones, particularly in the Rocky Mountain area. The prevalence rate obtained in this study was lower than the rate of 8.8 per 1000 found among military inductees (RuDusky, 1963). This difference may be due to the generally higher socio-economic status of college students.

A comparison of the recent college student survey to studies completed 20 to 30 years ago reveals a decline in the prevalence of rheumatic heart disease. Paul and Leddy (1932) and Cole (1941) reported rates of 8.2 and 8.0 per 1000 college student population. Despite this apparent decline the data obtained in this recent study indicate that rheumatic heart disease remains an important health problem in this country.

DECLINE IN SEVERITY OF RHEUMATIC FEVER

Residual Heart Disease

The change in severity can be judged by the decrease in cardiac involvement seen in patients hospitalized with acute rheumatic fever. Generally speaking the prognosis of any child is directly related to the severity of his carditis. Mayer et al. (1963) reported that among children discharged from the Bellevue Hospital the percentage of total cases with organic heart disease had decreased to 21 per cent between 1951 and 1958 as compared to 36.9 per cent for the preceding 16 years, 1935 to 1950. Massell et al. (1964) showed that among patients at The House of the Good Samaritan in Boston, the incidence of heart disease dropped from 73 per cent to 51 per cent in a comparison of two 10 year periods, 1921 to 1930 and 1951 to 1960.

Mortality

Mortality statistics also clearly reflect a change in severity. Death rates from acute rheumatic fever in all age groups have fallen from 16.8 per 100,000 population in 1910 to 0.4 in 1960 (Table 3). The death rate from rheumatic heart disease in children aged 5 to 14 years between 1920 and 1959 has shown a similar decrease (Table 4). The trend in mortality for the nonwhite differs from that of the white population. The death rate among white children has been declining steadily, whereas among the nonwhite population the rate increased until 1940 and since that time the rate has declined less than that for the whites.

Table 3.   Death Rates from Acute Rheumatic Fever
Per 100,000 Inhabitants

Year	Rate*
1900	14.3
1910	16.8
1920	10.3
1930	6.8
1940	3.5
1950	1.3
1960	0.4

* Corrected to reflect changes in coding rules according to Seventh Revision, International Lists of Causes of Deaths.

CAUSES OF THE CHANGING PATTERN OF RHEUMATIC FEVER

A number of factors have contributed to the decline in rheumatic fever. The widespread use of antimicrobial agents has undoubtedly reduced the spread of group A hemolytic streptococci, although infections with these organisms are still exceedingly common. There is no evidence to suggest that any fundamental change has occurred in the organism.

Table 4. Death Rates Per 100,000 Rheumatic Fever and Diseases of the Heart, U.S. Population, Ages 5 to 14 by Sex and Color, 1920-1959

Year	Cause of Death	Both Sexes All Races	White Male	White Female	Non-white Male	Non-white Female
1920	Acute RF*	4.4	4.3	4.7	2.4	3.2
	Heart diseases†	17.4	16.2	19.6	11.2	13.6
1930	Acute RF	3.0	3.0	3.0	2.8	3.3
	Heart diseases	12.1	11.2	12.9	12.8	11.6
1940	Acute RF	2.6	2.2	2.8	2.9	4.7
	Heart diseases	8.0	7.2	7.8	10.7	12.3
1950	Acute RF	1.8	1.4	1.8	2.9	4.6
	Heart diseases	2.1	1.7	1.9	3.4	4.3
1959	Acute RF	0.5	0.3	0.4	1.1	1.6
	Heart diseases	0.8	0.7	0.6	1.4	1.6

* RF = Rheumatic fever.
† All heart disease, including congenital and rheumatic.

Attack rates of rheumatic fever following epidemic streptococcal outbreaks have not changed. In 1926, an attack rate of 3.6 per cent was observed following a milk-borne outbreak of streptococcal infections in Denmark (Madsen, 1940). Twenty-five years later, a similar rate was reported by Rammelkamp and his co-workers (1952) among military recruits.

Mortality statistics indicate that the death rate from rheumatic fever and heart disease began to decrease before the advent of antimicrobial agents (Table 4). Living conditions were slowly improving during the 20 years before sulfonamides first became available in 1935. It was shown long ago in Denmark that slum clearance by itself will decrease the morbidity and mortality of rheumatic fever. In this country, in areas where housing conditions have not improved and poverty still exists, the decline in rheumatic fever has not been as striking. The incidence and severity of rheumatic fever remains high among Negro children living in slum areas. Similarly, rheumatic fever is common and severe among Puerto Rican children who have recently migrated to large northern cities and are living in substandard conditions. It is difficult to determine which environmental quality is the most significant. Crowding is undoubtedly an important factor since it predisposes to the rapid and repeated spread of streptococci from one person to another.

Continued improvement in social conditions is the major reason for the declining incidence of rheumatic fever. This trend has probably been accelerated by the use of antistreptococcal drugs. The chief role of antimicrobial agents, however, has been in the reduction in severe heart disease brought about by the introduction of continuous prophylaxis to prevent recurrent attacks. This is the chief reason why fewer patients with severe rheumatic heart disease are seen at the present time.

Despite this encouraging picture, it must be emphasized that rheumatic fever has far from disappeared. The incidence is undoubtedly still greater than is generally appreciated from available reports (Daugherty et al., 1963) and rheumatic fever is still the most common cause of acquired heart disease in individuals under 40 years of age (White, 1953). Experience in military camps during and after World War II indicates that sizable outbreaks of rheumatic fever can occur. Outbreaks may also occur occasionally in civilian communities. A recent example was reported in a small North Dakota community where 11 cases of rheumatic fever occurred among children in a three month period (Zimmerman et al., 1962).

Chapter Two

THE BIOLOGY OF GROUP
A BETA HEMOLYTIC
STREPTOCOCCI

The importance of group A streptococci in the etiology of rheumatic fever is well established. The progress that has been made both in the diagnosis and prevention of this disease during the past two decades is directly related to advances in our knowledge of the bacteriology of these organisms and of the immune response they evoke. The complexity of these bacteria can be appreciated from the list of many known cellular components and extracellular products shown in Table 5. This brief chapter reviews the structure and biologic characteristics of some of these substances which are relevant to the discussion of etiology and pathogenesis of rheumatic fever in the chapters which follow. The reader is

Table 5. Cellular Components and Extracellular Products of Group A Streptococci

Cellular Components	*Extracellular Products*
Hyaluronic acid (capsule)	Streptolysin O and S
Group-specific carbohydrate	Hyaluronidase
M, T, and R proteins	Streptokinase
Mucopeptide	Diphosphopyridine nucleotidase (DPNase)
Polyglycerophosphate	Deoxyribonucleases (DNase) A, B, C, and D
Beta glucuronidase	Erythrogenic toxin
Lipoproteinase	Proteinase
DNA, RNA	Ribonuclease
	Amylase

referred to several excellent monographs for a more comprehensive review (McCarty, 1954; Uhr, 1964).

CELLULAR COMPONENTS

The streptococcal cell is represented schematically in Figure 2. Virulent streptococci are usually surrounded by a capsule. The cell wall is made up of at least three distinct components, protein, carbohydrate, and mucopeptide (McCarty, 1964). When the cell wall is removed there remains a central core of cytoplasm which is surrounded by a distinct cytoplasmic membrane. The organisms from which the cell wall has been removed are called protoplasts.

The Capsule

The streptococcal capsule is composed of hyaluronate, a viscous mucopolysaccharide. It is not antigenic. Streptococcal hyaluronate is thought to be identical with the hyaluronate which is found in the connective tissues of man and animals. The failure to produce antibodies to streptococcal hyaluronate may be due to the wide distribution of hyaluronate in animal tissues (Lancefield, 1954). The capsule appears to be a factor in the virulence of group A streptococci, but its role seems to be relatively minor compared to that of the M protein, which will be dis-

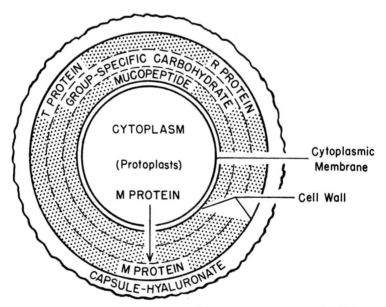

Figure 2. Schematic representation of a group A streptococcal cell (see text). (Modified from Krause, R. M.: Bact. Rev. 27:369, 1963.

cussed. At the present time there is no evidence that the capsular substance is involved in the pathogenesis of rheumatic fever.

Carbohydrate

The middle layer of the cell wall contains the carbohydrate component, and on the basis of this substance (group-specific polysaccharide) beta hemolytic streptococci can be separated into a number of serologically distinct groups. Each group is designated by the letters A to O. Over 90 per cent of human streptococcal infections are caused by one group designated as group A. Other groups such as C, D, G, and K may be involved occasionally in human infections but there is no evidence that infections with strains other than group A ever initiate an attack of rheumatic fever. The chemical composition of the group-specific carbohydrate has been defined (McCarty, 1964). It is weakly antigenic in man and antibodies against the group-specific C polysaccharide appear in the serum of only a small percentage of patients following an infection with Group A streptococci.

Protein

The outer surface layer of the cell wall contains three special proteins, the M, T, and R proteins, of which the M protein is the most important. The significance and properties of M protein have been comprehensively reviewed by Lancefield (1962). On the basis of the M protein, group A streptococci can be differentiated into distinct serologic types, numbered 1 to 50. In contrast to acute glomerulonephritis which is associated with only a few types, rheumatic fever may follow any one of the 50 known types. Virulence of group A streptococci depends chiefly on the presence of M protein which has antiphagocytic properties. The M protein of each type is the antigen which stimulates the formation of type-specific bactericidal antibodies. These antibodies confer long-lasting immunity, often for life, to the particular type causing the infection. Since they are type-specific, they do not protect against infections with other types. Thus, successive streptococcal infections in one person are each caused by a strain of a different serologic type. Unlike the antibodies evoked by streptococcal extracellular products, bactericidal antibodies to M protein appear in the circulation slowly, sometimes requiring several months before they can be detected. Formation of these antibodies is suppressed when the streptococcal infection is treated with antibiotics (Denny et al., 1957).

Mucopeptide

The inner layer of the streptococcal cell wall is a mucopeptide. Its chemical structure has been defined by Krause and McCarty (1961).

This substance is the skeletal component of the cell and is responsible for its shape and rigidity (McCarty, 1964). The morphologic integrity of the cell depends on the mucopeptide. Penicillin exerts its antibiotic effect by interfering with the biosynthesis of this substance.

Protoplasts

The cell wall can be removed from group A streptococci by several techniques, and such organisms from which the cell wall has been removed are called protoplasts. Protoplasts are probably identical with the so-called L forms, morphologic variants of the organisms which appear when streptococci are grown under special conditions. Streptococcal bacteriophage lysin may also convert streptococci to L forms. L forms are devoid of group-specific carbohydrate but still produce the M protein of the strain of group A streptococci from which they are derived (Sharp et al., 1957). L forms are penicillin resistant. Their possible role in the etiology of rheumatic fever is just beginning to be explored.

EXTRACELLULAR PRODUCTS

Group A streptococci secrete a number of substances into the surrounding culture media (Table 5). None of these substances, however, with the possible exception of streptolysin S, has been implicated in the pathogenesis of rheumatic fever. They are of importance, nevertheless, because with only one exception they are antigenic and evoke detectable antibodies in the sera of patients following a streptococcal infection. These antibodies may be measured by different methods and their presence is indicative of a recent streptococcal infection. Such evidence is often helpful in evaluating a patient in whom rheumatic fever is suspected. This discussion is limited to those extracellular substances which bear on the problems of rheumatic fever.

Streptolysin O

This enzyme hemolyzes red blood cells and is termed streptolysin O because it is oxygen labile and therefore is inactive on the surface of blood agar plates. It has been shown to possess toxicity not only for erythrocytes but for the amphibian heart as well. It is a potent antigen and elicits an antibody response in 70 to 85 per cent of patients following an infection with group A streptococci. Antibody against streptolysin O (antistreptolysin O, or ASO) is the most commonly measured antibody because it can be easily quantitated. Antibodies to streptolysin O can usually be demonstrated one week after a streptococcal infection and the maximum level is reached in 3 to 5 weeks. Prompt penicillin treatment of a streptococcal infection may suppress the ASO response.

Streptolysin S

The second hemolysin produced by group A streptococci is termed streptolysin S because it is obtained by extraction of organisms with animal sera. This hemolysin is responsible for the zone of hemolysis which surrounds colonies of beta streptococci growing on the surface of blood agar plates. Streptolysin S is nonantigenic and is inhibited by normal human sera. Its possible significance in the pathogenesis of rheumatic fever is discussed in the next chapter.

Streptokinase

Tillett and Garner (1933) were the first to report that culture filtrates of beta streptococci liquefied fibrin clots. It is now known that the streptococcal enzyme, streptokinase, converts a normal serum component, plasminogen, to an active proteolytic enzyme, plasmin. Streptokinase is antigenic and methods are available for assaying antistreptokinase antibody levels. In general, following a streptococcal infection, a rise in antistreptokinase titer occurs less frequently than a rise in the ASO level. In addition, antistreptokinase determinations are difficult to standardize and for these reasons this antibody test is not generally used.

Hyaluronidase

The enzyme depolymerizes hyaluronic acid. Only two of the 50 types of group A streptococci (types 4 and 22) produce large amounts of hyaluronidase in vitro. The small amounts of this enzyme formed by the other types are, however, antigenically potent, and stimulate the production of antihyaluronidase antibodies. The response is similar to that observed with antistreptolysin O. Some investigators have suggested that in patients with rheumatic fever the antibody response to hyaluronidase is greater than that of other streptococcal antigens (Harris and Harris, 1950). There has been some difficulty in standardizing the method for determining antihyaluronidase antibodies, but satisfactory test materials have recently become commercially available.

Diphosphopyridine Nucleotidase (DPNase)

This streptococcal enzyme splits DPN and was first reported by Carlson et al. (1957). These investigators also demonstrated that this enzyme is antigenic (Kellner et al., 1958). Bernhard and Stollerman (1959) found a significant rise in antibody (anti-DPNase) in 87 per cent of patients with acute rheumatic fever, equal to the percentage of patients with an elevated ASO titer. Ayoub and Wannamaker (1962) observed that anti-DPNase titers tended to be higher in patients with acute nephritis than in those with acute rheumatic fever. Accurate methods are available for the determination of anti-DPNase levels and it has been recommended as one of the more useful streptococcal antibody tests (Wannamaker and Ayoub, 1960).

Deoxyribonucleases (DNase)

Streptococci produce extracellular enzymes which depolymerize deoxyribonucleic acid (DNA) (Tillett et al., 1948; McCarty, 1948). Wannamaker (1958, 1962) has shown that group A streptococci produce four immunologically distinct deoxyribonucleases which have been designated DNase A, B, C, and D. Each of these DNases evokes specific antibodies. Group A streptococci produce DNase B in the largest quantities and in general the antibody response to this antigen is the most consistent of the DNases. Ayoub and Wannamaker (1962) have shown that the rise in anti-DNase B titers in patients with acute rheumatic fever is comparable to the antistreptolysin O response. They have suggested that the anti-DNase B determination is a useful secondary test in patients suspected of having rheumatic fever and in whom the ASO titer is low or equivocal. These investigators have also found that the anti-DNase titer remains elevated longer than the ASO titer and have suggested that this antibody test may prove valuable in patients with chorea in whom there is often a long interval between the streptococcal infection and the rheumatic attack (Wannamaker, 1964). At the present time, however, the usefulness of the anti-DNase B test is somewhat limited by difficulties in preparing a satisfactory enzyme.

Chapter Three

ETIOLOGY

THE RELATIONSHIP OF GROUP A STREPTOCOCCI
TO RHEUMATIC FEVER

Our understanding of the role played by group A hemolytic strepto-cocci in rheumatic fever is based on data accumulated over many years in various fields of investigation: clinical, immunologic, epidemiologic, and prophylactic. Confirmatory evidence is constantly being added, and some of the more recent findings will be included in this discussion of etiology and in the chapter on pathogenesis which follows.

Clinical Studies

One hundred years ago clinicians noted that endocarditis, arthritis, and chorea often followed scarlet fever (Trousseau, 1865). It was recog-nized subsequently that rheumatic fever could also follow tonsillitis and septic sore throat. In 1886, Haig-Brown introduced the concept of the latent period between the sore throat and the onset of rheumatic symp-toms. Because of the sporadic occurrence of rheumatic fever in the general population, the relationship between this disease and throat infections was not generally accepted for many decades. However, in 1930 to 1932 a number of investigators reported that in closed communities, such as boarding schools and convalescent homes for rheumatic children, multiple cases of rheumatic fever occurred following outbreaks of scarlet fever or tonsillitis (Schlesinger, 1930; Collis, 1931; Coburn, 1931). Thus the observations previously recorded in individual patients were confirmed by epidemiologic studies.

The medical profession, nevertheless, remained dubious of the rela-

15

tionship of throat infections and rheumatic fever. The variety of bacteria
implicated as causative agents resulted in considerable confusion. At that
time the techniques for the identification and classification of streptococci
were not sufficiently developed to establish the role of these organisms in
human disease. Subsequently Lancefield (1940) differentiated hemolytic
streptococci into a number of distinct groups and demonstrated that a
special group, designated group A, was the chief cause of streptococcal
infections in man. Thus it became established that scarlet fever and septic
sore throat were due to group A hemolytic streptococci, and that in some
individuals these infections were followed by rheumatic fever. It is now
recognized that rheumatic fever may also follow mild or inapparent
streptococcal infections. Since rheumatic fever is known to be a sequel
of streptococcal pharyngitis, the importance of recognizing streptococcal
illnesses and of instituting adequate treatment is generally recognized.

Immunologic Studies

In 1932 Todd developed a method for measuring an antibody directed
against a streptococcal hemolysin (streptolysin O). This test made it
possible to obtain immunologic evidence of a streptococcal infection and
it was particularly useful in patients who did not have a history of a sore
throat or scarlet fever. Indeed, at least 50 per cent of patients with rheumatic fever do not have a history of a preceding illness. Moreover, the
throat culture is frequently negative for beta hemolytic streptococci at
the time the rheumatic symptoms appear. For these reasons Todd's con-
tribution was of enormous importance in establishing the relationship
between streptococcal infections and rheumatic fever.

As noted in the previous chapter, group A streptococci produce a
number of extracellular antigens in addition to streptolysin O, such as
streptokinase, hyaluronidase, deoxyribonuclease, and diphosphopyridine
nucleotidase. Each of these antigens evokes specific antibodies in human
sera but not all patients respond uniformly to each antigen. For example,
15 to 20 percent of patients with acute rheumatic fever do not have an
elevated ASO titer. In such children, the occurrence of a preceding streptococcal infection can be established by a study of antibodies to one of the
other streptococcal antigens mentioned. If the sera of patients with acute
rheumatic fever are examined for at least three streptococcal antibodies,
evidence of a recent streptococcal infection can be obtained in 95 per
cent (Stollerman et al., 1956).

In general, antibodies to extracellular antigens begin to rise 7 to 10
days after a streptococcal infection and reach their peak in 3 to 5 weeks.
The antibody response is quantitatively greater in patients who develop
rheumatic fever than in patients with uncomplicated streptococcal infections. However, there is so much variation in antibody titers that the
magnitude of the rise is not of itself of diagnostic value. The titers return

to normal levels in 2 to 4 months and for this reason, streptococcal anti-body titers are usually normal in the chronic stage of rheumatic disease.

Epidemiologic Studies

It has already been noted that studies of outbreaks of rheumatic fever in closed communities carried out several decades ago provided important epidemiologic evidence for the role of the streptococcus in rheumatic fever. Further evidence came from careful studies of outbreaks of streptococcal infections and rheumatic fever in military training centers during and following World War II (Rammelkamp et al., 1952). An example of the relationship between an epidemic of streptococcal infections and rheumatic fever in a naval training center is shown in Figure 3.

Studies of rheumatic fever in military populations have shown a fairly constant attack rate of 3 per cent following untreated epidemic streptococcal infections (Rammelkamp et al., 1952). Such epidemics are usually due to the spread of group A streptococci of one or two types rich in M protein. Infections with these organisms cause definite clinical signs and symptoms characterized by pharyngeal exudate, fever, and an elevated white blood count. A high ASO titer and prolonged carriage of the

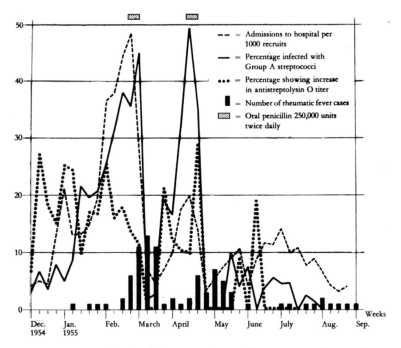

Figure 3. An outbreak of rheumatic fever following an epidemic of group A streptococcal infection at a naval recruit training center. (Courtesy Naval Medical Research Unit No. 4, Great Lakes Naval Training Center.)

organism are more likely following infection with an epidemic strain. Rheumatic fever occurs more commonly in such patients.

In contrast to the high incidence of rheumatic fever observed in epidemics of streptococcal pharyngitis, the attack rate is much lower following endemic or sporadic streptococcal upper respiratory infections usually seen in the civilian population. Among 519 untreated children with signs or symptoms of sore throat seen in an outpatient department of a Chicago hospital, Siegel and his co-workers (1961) reported that only two patients developed rheumatic fever, an attack rate of 0.33 per cent, approximately one-tenth of that observed under epidemic conditions. All 519 children harbored group A streptococci, but in the majority of patients the pharyngitis was mild, and no exudate was present. Convalescent carriage of the organism occurred infrequently. Forty-eight per cent of the strains isolated were deficient in M antigen and could not be typed. Only 45 per cent of the patients developed a significant rise in ASO titer. These findings suggest that milder streptococcal disease is associated with relatively low rheumatic attack rates. Similar results have been obtained in other studies (Goslings et al., 1963). However, when streptococcal infections of an epidemic nature occur in civilian populations, the attack rate of rheumatic fever may be high. For example, an outbreak of group A streptococcal infections in an isolated North Dakota community resulted in 11 cases of rheumatic fever among school children over a period of 8 weeks (Zimmerman et al., 1962).

Studies of Prophylactic Treatment

Chemotherapeutic agents that could effectively prevent beta hemolytic streptococcal infections became available in 1936. Because of the high recurrence rate of rheumatic fever, daily oral doses of sulfonamides were tried as a prophylactic measure to prevent streptococcal infections in rheumatic subjects in convalescent homes and in pediatric cardiac clinics. Well controlled studies showed that by this procedure streptococcal upper respiratory infections could be prevented and that the recurrence rate of rheumatic fever was greatly reduced. Subsequently, similar results were obtained with daily oral doses of penicillin.

In the general population the incidence of initial attacks of rheumatic fever is low. Adequate data based on large numbers of patients with streptococcal infections were needed to prove that first attacks of rheumatic fever could be prevented by penicillin therapy. During an epidemic of streptococcal pharyngitis in a military training center, Rammelkamp and his co-workers (Denny et al., 1950) treated 798 patients with exudative tonsillitis with penicillin. In this group only two cases of rheumatic fever occurred whereas in a similar group of 804 untreated recruits there were 17 cases of rheumatic fever. As a result of these findings, it is now established that the administration of adequate doses of penicillin for 10 days to children with scarlet fever or streptococcal pharyngitis may prevent the appearance of rheumatic fever. Treatment for a full 10 day period is essential to eliminate streptococci from the nasopharynx. If antibiotics are given for only a few days, these organisms may reappear in the throat and rheumatic fever may develop.

The demonstration that prevention and treatment of streptococcal infections reduced the incidence of rheumatic fever provided striking additional evidence that group A streptococci play an important role in the etiology of rheumatic fever.

PREDISPOSING FACTORS

Although streptococcal infections are very common in man, only a very small percentage of individuals develop rheumatic fever. Additional factors are undoubtedly involved. Inherited or acquired differences in the host, environmental conditions, or a combination may be important determinants. These aspects of rheumatic fever have been less well studied than the inciting organism, chiefly because they are more difficult to assess in a disease which occurs so sporadically and which is so variable. Nevertheless the ecology of rheumatic fever, although poorly understood, is of considerable importance. To paraphrase Galdston (1957), there may be more to learn from the *man* sick than from the man's *sickness*.

Host Characteristics

Genetic Factors. Cheadle (1889), 75 years ago, was the first to record that rheumatic fever frequently occurred in more than one member of the family. Numerous studies have since confirmed the high family incidence of this disease. A larger percentage of children born of rheumatic parents contract the disease than of those born of nonrheumatic parents. The incidence is also higher in relatives of rheumatic children who live in separate households than among relatives of nonrheumatic children.

Many studies have sought to explain the basis for this familial tendency. Extensive investigations by Wilson et al. (1943, 1954) in a large number of rheumatic families led these workers to conclude that rheumatic susceptibility is based on a single autosomal recessive gene. This view has been confirmed by some investigators (Mallen and Castillo, 1952), but not by others (Gray, 1952; Stevenson and Cheeseman, 1953, 1956). Stevenson and Cheeseman studied 2038 children of 462 families and found that although inheritance appeared to play an important role in rheumatic fever, it did not follow a Mendelian pattern. Taranta and co-workers (1959) studied 56 rheumatic fever patients and their co-twins. Of 16 pairs who were monozygotic, 3 were concordant for rheumatic fever and the type of rheumatic manifestation. Of 40 sets of twins who were dizygotic, 2 pairs were concordant for rheumatic fever. These authors concluded that since less than one-fifth of the monozygotic twins were concordant for rheumatic fever, genetic factors have only limited penetrance.

Blood groups and secretor status of rheumatic subjects have been studied in an attempt to identify a susceptible genotype. Glynn and his associates (1959) studied the secretion of blood group substances of a large number of rheumatic patients. They found a higher incidence of ABO nonsecretors in rheumatic subjects than among healthy school children, but the observed differences were too small to warrant conclusions (Glynn et al., 1961). Other investigators have found a lower frequency of blood group O in rheumatic children, but the significance of this finding is not clear (Clarke et al., 1960).

Although it is stated at times that rheumatic fever is more common among girls, available data do not show any significant sex differences except in patients with chorea. Females are more likely to have chorea than are males. There are sex differences in the type of valvular lesions. In adults, mitral stenosis is more common in females but males have a higher incidence of aortic regurgitation.

The roles of streptococcus and of environmental factors in the high family incidence of rheumatic fever are not fully understood. Environmental conditions which predispose to the spread of streptococcal infections through a family may also increase susceptibility to rheumatic fever. In a study of a communal settlement with a high prevalence of rheumatic heart disease and a high incidence of streptococcal infections, Davies and Lazarov (1960) found that children from families in which one or both parents had rheumatic heart disease were more susceptible to streptococcal infections than controls with identical exposure. Unpublished observations from the Johns Hopkins Rheumatic Fever Clinic suggest that the siblings of rheumatic children do not have an increased susceptibility to streptococcal infections nor an unusual immune response following such infections. It is unusual for 2 cases of rheumatic fever in a family to occur simultaneously. A child may have pharyngitis due to the same type of streptococcus as the one which caused the attack in his sibling without developing rheumatic fever. However, following pharyngitis due to a streptococcus of a different type rheumatic fever may occur.

Knowledge of genetic factors in rheumatic fever is incomplete. It is generally agreed that there is an inherited susceptibility but the mode of inheritance and the methods of its expression are not clear. It is likely that heredity and environment are both involved in the high familial incidence. In the absence of an index case, rheumatic families have no known characteristics by which they can be identified. In known rheumatic families, however, the physician should be aware that streptococcal pharyngitis represents a special hazard and, therefore, it is advisable to take throat cultures whenever upper respiratory infections occur.

Race and Ethnic Groups. It has been suggested that rheumatic fever occurs more commonly in certain ethnic groups. Earlier in this century, the Irish were considered particularly prone to this disease (Coburn, 1931; Stroud and Twaddle, 1940), and Negroes were less susceptible. A high incidence of rheumatic fever occurs in any ethnic group which recently has migrated to cities where housing is inadequate and the number of persons per room is excessive. There are no valid data which show differences in susceptibility on the basis of race or ethnic group (Wilson, 1940; Diamond, 1959). Although living conditions appear to be the chief determinant in the differences which have been observed, other environmental factors, such as a change in climate or altitude, possibly play a part.

Age. Rheumatic fever is uncommon in children less than 5 years of age and is rarely seen under the age of 2. Hedley (1940) reported that 0.7 per cent of 2324 patients had their initial attack under 2 years of age and only 8.4 per cent under the age of 5 years. The greatest incidence occurs between 6 and 15 years with a peak at about 8 years.

This age distribution coincides in part with the recognized high incidence of streptococcal infections in school-age children. Streptococcal infections, however, are also encountered frequently in the preschool child. In a clinical and bacteriologic study of upper respiratory illnesses in a pediatric population, 40 per cent of the streptococcal infections occurred in children 2 to 6 years of age (Markowitz, 1963A). In this age group the incidence of rheumatic fever is low compared to the frequency of streptococcal infections. Rantz and his colleagues (1945) suggested that the greater susceptibility to rheumatic fever after 6 years of age was the result of repeated streptococcal infections. Furthermore, these investigators showed that the antistreptolysin O response following a streptococcal infection increases from infancy through childhood and theorized that this was due to a changing pattern with age in the host's immune response (Rantz et al., 1951). Their hypothesis implied that rheumatic subjects had a greater number of streptococcal infections than nonrheumatic individuals. However, data obtained in a recent study do not support this theory (Markowitz, 1963B). On the basis of type-specific antibody determinations, this investigator could find no evidence to indicate that rheumatic individuals had a greater number of streptococcal infections before the infection which triggered that attack than nonrheumatic children. These studies do not exclude the possibility that the host's response is changed in some manner by age, but it seems unlikely that the number of previous streptococcal infections is the critical factor.

The incidence of initial attacks of rheumatic fever decreases after puberty, probably because exposure to streptococcal infection decreases during adolescence and adult life. Experience in the Armed Forces, however, demonstrates clearly that when young adults are exposed to virulent streptococcal infections, the incidence of rheumatic fever is high. At the Naval Training Center in Farragut, Idaho, the attack rate of rheumatic fever in 1943 was 37.8 per 1000 personnel (Coburn and Young, 1949). It has also been shown that susceptibility to rheumatic recurrences remains relatively high until at least 22 years of age (Johnson et al., 1964).

Nutrition. A deficient diet is often associated with poverty and although the prevalence of rheumatic fever is higher among the poor, there is no evidence to indicate a predisposing dietary deficiency of a specific nature. Coburn (1960) has suggested that diet may indeed play a specific role and that substances such as phospholipids may be involved in the etiology of rheumatic fever. No data are available to support this view. Although anemia occurs with active rheumatic fever, it is not present prior to the onset of the attack. Indeed, rheumatic fever is remarkably uncommon in children with chronic anemia associated with sickle cell disease.

Emotional Factors. There has been considerable interest in the relationship of emotional stress as a factor in susceptibility to disease. However very little attention has been paid to the emotional health of the families of rheumatic children. Grave (1957), in a study of social and environmental factors in the etiology of rheumatic fever, attempted to assess certain emotional factors and found that a higher percentage of children with rheumatic fever had a disturbed mother-child relationship than did a control group. However, the differences were not pronounced and they could not be separated from other factors.

Recently Meyer and Haggerty (1962) studied factors related to susceptibility of streptococcal infections in families. These observers found that the occurrence of such infections was significantly greater in families under conditions of acute as well as chronic stress. The number of patients studied was too small to judge the incidence of rheumatic fever, but any factor which increases the streptococcal attack rate is likely to increase the frequency of this complication.

Adrenocortical Function. Interest in the role of steroids in rheumatic fever stimulated the investigation of adrenocortical function in rheumatic subjects. On the basis of studies of circulating hydroxycorticoid steroid levels in rheumatic and nonrheumatic children, Kelley (1955) suggested that there may be a relative adrenal insufficiency in rheumatic patients. More recently these same investigators have stated that although adrenal function and steroid metabolism are not completely normal in rheumatic subjects, the differences are difficult to demonstrate, and that there is no evidence to suggest that these abnormalities are related to the pathogenesis of rheumatic fever (Kelley and Ely, 1960).

Environmental Factors

Socio-economic. Rheumatic fever occurs among all levels of society. It is, however, more common and even more strikingly severe in children who endure substandard living conditions.

A number of investigations have been carried out to ascertain the importance of social and environmental conditions associated with rheumatic fever. Many of these studies have been reviewed by Paul (1957). Crowding, poor hygiene, substandard housing, and inadequate medical care all favor the spread of streptococcal infections and probably influence the attack rate of rheumatic fever in this manner. Of these factors, crowding may be the most significant. It has obvious implications in the epidemiology of streptococcal infections and may well account for the higher attack rate of rheumatic fever in urban areas, slums, and large families. Several studies have shown a significant correlation between crowding and the prevalence of rheumatic fever and rheumatic heart disease (Perry and Roberts, 1937; Clarke, 1940; Quinn et al., 1950). However, Diamond (1957) evaluated environmental conditions which might influence the attack rate and found that when each factor was considered separately no difference could be found, although a combination of these factors did influence the incidence of this disease. It is likely that the circumstances which attend poverty not only favor the spread of streptococci but diminish the resistance to streptococcal infections, as well as to tuberculosis and other illnesses.

There is much truth in the statement that "rheumatic fever is a social ailment" (Stamler, 1962). The decline in frequency and severity generally noted in the United States has been less striking where poverty still exists. It is well to recall that much of the improvement in rheumatic fever morbidity and mortality antedated antimicrobial agents and although drug prophylaxis is important, continued improvement of living conditions ("biologic prophylaxis") may be of even greater importance.

Climate and Geography. Rheumatic fever is a worldwide disease and its frequency appears to be influenced by climate and geography. Although most prevalent in the temperate zones, it is more common in tropical climates than was formerly supposed. Mortality figures indicate that death rates from rheumatic heart disease are lower in the southern states (Paul, 1947) and these data suggest that the disease is milder in these areas.

Studies of the incidence of streptococcal infections and rheumatic fever in one southern area (Miami, Florida) have been carried out by Saslaw and his co-workers (1959, 1960). These investigators found that streptococci are frequently present in the throats of Miami children. The incidence of rheumatic fever and rheumatic heart disease, however, was low. Although these observers found that a rise in the antistreptolysin O titer occurred in 50 per cent of the children, the maximal levels of antistreptolysin O were not as high as those commonly observed in the North. These findings suggest that streptococcal disease in Miami may be less potent antigenically and therefore causes a lower incidence of rheumatic fever (Stollerman, 1961).

The attack rate of rheumatic fever increases at high altitudes. In the United States, the high incidence of rheumatic fever in the Rocky Mountain states is striking (see Fig. 1). Rheumatic heart disease is prevalent in Mexico City, altitude 6000 feet (Chavez, 1942). Brand-Auraban (1959) found an unusually high incidence of acute rheumatic fever (6.5 per 1000) in Jerusalem, which is well above sea level as compared to the incidence in the coastal areas (1.5 per 1000). The meteorologic conditions associated with high altitudes, such as coldness and dryness, may be important.

Season. There is a definite seasonal incidence of rheumatic fever which varies in different localities. On the west coast of the United States, the peak is usually reached in January and February, along the eastern seaboard in March and April, and in England in November. In general the seasonal variation in rheumatic fever follows that of streptococcal disease.

THE LATENT PERIOD

The sequence of events following streptococcal upper respiratory infections was carefully documented by Coburn in 1931. Both the initial attack of rheumatic fever and recurrences in known rheumatic subjects follow a characteristic pattern. The streptococcal pharyngitis, designated as *phase I*, may be moderately severe, mild, or subclinical so that it is recognized only by a rise in titer of streptococcal antibodies. When clinical symptoms are present, they usually subside in 3 or 4 days if no suppurative complication supervenes. The patient then appears well for a period of time. This asymptomatic or latent period is designated as *phase II*. The latent period or phase II is followed by appearance of acute rheumatic fever, designated as *phase III*.

It has been possible to measure the length of the latent period only in rheumatic patients with a history of a sore throat. Such a history can be obtained usually in about 50 per cent of the patients. The length of the latent period is variable. The most accurate study has been carried out by Rammelkamp and Stolzer (1961) on 251 patients in whom the streptococcal pharyngitis was observed prior to the onset of acute rheumatic fever. In the majority of patients the latent period was between 1 and 3 weeks. Twenty-four per cent showed latent periods of over 35 days. However in a number of patients with long latent periods, reinfection with a different type of streptococcus was demonstrated. Seven per cent of the patients had a latent period of less than 5 days and in 2 patients the symptoms of acute rheumatic fever coincided with the onset of the respiratory illness. The length of the latent period does not appear to be related to the specific type of group A streptococci isolated from the throat, the height of the streptococcal antibody titer, or the clinical pattern of the rheumatic episode.

Little is known of what occurs in the host during the latent period. Rantz and co-workers (1945) suggested that reinfection with a new serologic type during the latent period might be related to the development of acute rheumatic fever. However, data published by Stetson (1954) do not support the view that closely spaced infections play a causative role in rheumatic fever. The latent period has been compared to the interval observed in serum sickness after the injection of a potent antigen. However, there is no evidence to indicate that the latent period is shortened during a rheumatic recurrence similar to the accelerated reaction seen in serum sickness disease following the readministration of the responsible antigen. Studies of the host during the latent period have not yet yielded any clues concerning the pathogenesis of rheumatic fever.

Chapter Four

PATHOGENESIS

There is no longer any doubt that rheumatic fever is a sequel to a group A streptococcal infection. However, the mechanism by which these organisms precipitate rheumatic fever in susceptible individuals is still not understood. Many attempts have been made to elucidate the role of group A hemolytic streptococci in the pathogenesis of rheumatic fever. In general these studies have been directed to answer the following questions: (1) Is rheumatic fever the result of the persistence of streptococci or variants of these organisms? (2) Are the lesions of rheumatic fever caused by streptococcal toxins or enzymes? (3) Is rheumatic fever a hypersensitivity or an auto-immune disorder? (4) Can rheumatic fever be induced experimentally?

IS RHEUMATIC FEVER THE RESULT OF THE PERSISTENCE OF STREPTOCOCCI OR VARIANTS OF THESE ORGANISMS?

Rheumatic fever does not have the clinical features of a bacterial infection and streptococci are not generally demonstrable in the lesions. The usual inflammatory reaction caused by the direct invasion of bacteria does not occur in the cardiac, joint, or brain tissues of rheumatic patients. For these reasons physicians were reluctant for many years to accept the idea that rheumatic fever was precipitated by a streptococcal throat infection. The possible persistence of viable streptococci has remained an attractive hypothesis since it could explain the intense immune response to streptococcal antigens noted in rheumatic patients and might account for the prolonged activity of the rheumatic process in some patients.

In 1939 and 1940, several investigators reported independently that they had isolated group A streptococci from cultures of affected heart valves from patients dying of rheumatic fever (Green, 1939; Collis, 1939; Thomson and Innes, 1940). Both Green and Thomson and Innes found that the streptococci isolated were of the same serologic type as those recovered from the nasopharynx of the patients before death and were therefore probably not contaminants.

The observations reported by these investigators did not receive much attention until studies on the prevention of rheumatic fever with penicillin by Rammelkamp and his associates suggested that the persistence of living streptococci might be important in the pathogenesis of rheumatic fever. Rammelkamp and his co-workers (Denny et al., 1950) found that it was essential to use penicillin in amounts sufficient to eradicate completely the organisms from the nasopharynx in order to prevent rheumatic fever effectively. Further studies by this group of investigators (Catanzaro et al., 1954) showed that rheumatic fever could be prevented by the administration of penicillin even as late as 9 days after streptococcal pharyngitis. On the other hand, sulfonamides did not reduce the rheumatic fever attack rate because these agents did not always eradicate the organisms completely.

Mortimer et al. (1959) also studied the possibility that rheumatic fever might represent a form of group A streptococcal endocarditis. Ninety-seven patients with acute rheumatic fever were divided into two groups: 49 received massive penicillin therapy for 6 weeks and 48 were given no antimicrobial medication. No difference was observed in the response of the clinical or laboratory manifestations during the acute stage. However, these investigators found that one year after completion of treatment, there was a significant reduction in the incidence of heart disease in the penicillin group. They concluded that their results were consistent with the possibility that living streptococci play a role in the development of valvular heart disease even after symptoms of rheumatic fever appear.

It is the impression of most observers that the conclusions drawn by Mortimer et al. were not justified on the basis of the data presented and that further studies are needed. Furthermore, an investigation carried out by Watson et al. (1961), which was done before penicillin was available but which was published only recently, did not confirm the postmortem bacteriologic findings reported by the British pathologists. Watson and his associates found that microorganisms could not be cultured from the heart valves when strict aseptic precautions were used at the autopsy table.

Although at the present time there is no conclusive evidence that the persistence of group A streptococci is involved in the pathogenesis of rheumatic fever, the possibility that streptococci are present as L forms has not been excluded. One of the striking characteristics of L forms is their ability to survive in the presence of penicillin. The L form is a small globule, not much larger than some of the viruses, and Maxted (1964) has suggested the possibility that they may penetrate and survive in cells for long periods of time much as some viruses do. Wittler et al. (1962) have reported that transitional forms of streptococci which may be related to L forms were cultured from the blood of patients with rheumatic fever and Kagan (1962) has reported similar findings. However, these observations need confirmation. Further investigations of L forms are now in progress.

ARE THE LESIONS OF RHEUMATIC FEVER CAUSED BY STREPTOCOCCAL TOXINS OR ENZYMES?

The cellular components and extracellular products of group A streptococci have been reviewed in Chapter 2 and, as has been noted, much has been learned regarding these substances. Although it has not been possible to prove that any one of them is the cause of rheumatic fever, several recent studies are of interest.

The group-specific polysaccharide contained within the cell wall of group A streptococci has been implicated as a cause of connective tissue lesions in animals. Schwab and Cromartie (1957) and Cromartie (1964) have described chronic nodular lesions produced by sonically disrupted group A streptococci injected intradermally into rabbits. These investigators consider these lesions to be due to the group-specific polysaccharide contained in these preparations. McCarty (1964) however, doubts that these toxic reactions are due primarily to this substance, since a similar reaction occurs with preparations of group C streptococci.

Streptococcal extracellular products are enzymes which differ greatly in biologic activity and are produced in varying amounts by all types of group A streptococci. During the course of streptococcal infections specific antibodies to some or all of these enzymes develop and inhibit their activity. After recovery, the titers of these antibodies return to normal levels, but in every subsequent streptococcal upper respiratory infection these antibodies are produced again, usually more rapidly and in greater quantity (accelerated secondary response). Potent as these streptococcal enzymes are against their specific substrates (erythrocytes, hyaluronic acid, fibrin, DNA, and others) their activities in vivo are probably neutralized, and there is no proof that they cause serious tissue injury.

In contrast to the majority of extracellular substances, streptolysin S is not antigenic. It is a toxic substance which causes myocardial necrosis in mice. Todd and his co-workers (1939) found that sera from patients with acute rheumatic fever tended to inhibit streptolysin S less than sera from inactive rheumatic subjects. Stollerman and Bernheimer (1950) confirmed these observations but the significance of this finding is not clear.

Recently the work of Hirschhorn and associates (1964) has given renewed emphasis to the possible role of streptolysin S in rheumatic fever. These investigators found that streptolysin S added to cultures of lymphocytes from normal individuals transformed these cells into large lymphocytes and plasma cells, but failed to do so when added to the cell cultures of lymphocytes obtained from patients with acute rheumatic fever. They also showed that the lymphocytes again responded normally after the rheumatic patients were treated with penicillin. These observers suggest that patients with rheumatic fever are unable to neutralize streptolysin S. Since streptolysin S is not antigenic and is therefore not specifically inhibited by antibody, this enzyme would be free to cause tissue damage. Further studies are needed to explore this hypothesis.

Zabriskie (1964) has investigated the relationship of streptococcal bacteriophage to the production of the erythrogenic streptococcal exotoxin which causes the characteristic rash of scarlet fever. He has shown that lysogenic strains of group A streptococci infected with a bacterial virus (bacteriophage) produce this toxin but noninfected strains do not. Zabriskie's findings are comparable to the results of the earlier classic studies of Freeman (1951) who demonstrated that when avirulent strains of C diphtheriae were rendered lysogenic by bacteriophage, they produced diphtheria toxin. Kjems (1955) and Krause (1957) have reported that lysogenic strains are common among group A hemolytic streptococci and that during the course of an epidemic there may be a change from non-lysogenic to lysogenic strains (Kjems, 1960). It has also been shown that bacteriophage lysin can convert streptococci to L forms (Freimer et al. 1959). It is possible that phage-induced changes in streptococci may make these organisms "rheumatogenic" through the production of a specific toxin substance or by the induction of streptococcal L forms in the human body. The latter possibility will become particularly attractive if it is confirmed that L forms can be recovered from blood cultures of rheumatic subjects.

IS RHEUMATIC FEVER A HYPERSENSITIVITY OR AN AUTO-IMMUNE DISEASE?

The possibility that rheumatic fever is due to a hypersensitivity reaction has been under consideration for many years because rheumatic fever in many ways resembles serum sickness (Klinge, 1933). Rheumatic fever, like serum sickness, can be divided into three phases: phase I, the streptococcal infections; phase II, the asymptomatic latent period during which antibodies are produced; and phase III, the period of active rheumatic fever. There are many histologic and clinical similarities between serum sickness and rheumatic fever. Hypersensitivity reactions produced in experimental animals by a variety of methods cause lesions which resemble those observed in rheumatic fever. The role of hypersensitivity in the pathogenesis of rheumatic fever has been reviewed by McCarty (1956) and MacLeod (1959).

It has been observed repeatedly that patients who develop rheumatic fever have a greater elevation in mean streptococcal antibody titers than nonrheumatic individuals with uncomplicated streptococcal infections. This exaggerated streptococcal antibody response was also in accord with the concept that an antigen-antibody reaction might play a significant role. The possibility that rheumatic subjects might be immunologically hyperreactive not only to streptococcal but also to heterologous antigens has been extensively investigated. The response to bacterial (typhoid vaccine, *Brucella abortus*), viral (influenza), polysaccharide (pneumococci), and toxoid (diphtheria) antigens in rheumatic and nonrheumatic children has been compared. With the exception of *Brucella abortus* no significant difference between normal and rheumatic individuals was observed. Wagner and Rejholec (1955) reported that with *Brucella abortus* higher titers of incomplete antibodies were obtained in rheumatic subjects than in controls. However, Kuhns and McCarty (1954), following the injection of diphtheria toxoid, found no difference in incomplete antibodies between rheumatic and nonrheumatic children. Studies of the antibody response of rheumatic children following injections of concentrates of streptolysin O suggest that these children show greater ASO responses than nonrheumatic children (Quinn et al., 1957). However, 5 of 20 rheumatic children studied showed no detectable antibody response. At the present time there are no valid data to indicate that the immune response of rheumatic patients differs significantly from that of normal individuals.

A series of investigations by Kaplan (1963) has introduced a new approach to the study of immunologic mechanisms in the pathogenesis of rheumatic fever. This investigator reported an interesting finding which suggests a definite relationship between group A streptococci and the myocardium. He has demonstrated that these organisms and normal human myocardial fiber share a common antigen (cross-reactive antigen) which thus far has not been identified with any of the known protein constituents of the streptococcal cell. Zabriskie (1964) has reported that this antigen is present in the cytoplasmic membrane of the streptococcal cell and not in the cell wall. When the sera of rheumatic patients as well as sera of rabbits immunized with group A streptococci are added to preparations of normal human myocardium, an antigen-antibody reaction develops along the myocardial fibers. Studies by Kaplan et al. (1961) using immunofluorescent techniques have shown that the sera of patients with active rheumatic fever frequently contain antibodies to this cross-reactive antigen. Hess and her associates (1964) found that 63.4 per cent of 171 patients with active rheumatic carditis had antibodies which reacted with human heart muscle as compared to 16.4 per cent of a group of inactive rheumatic subjects. These studies suggest that rheumatic fever may be an auto-immune disease. However, it is possible that the circulating auto-antibodies which have been demonstrated are the result rather than the cause of tissue damage. The concept that rheumatic fever is due to a hypersensitivity reaction to group A streptococci has not been established, nor can this disease be classified at the present time as an auto-immune disorder on the basis of available data.

CAN RHEUMATIC FEVER BE INDUCED EXPERIMENTALLY?

Antigen-antibody reactions of the Arthus type induced in animals by the injection of bacterial or protein antigens have been studied by a number of investigators in an attempt to reproduce the lesions of rheumatic fever. Rich (1946) injected rabbits intravenously with large quantities of horse serum and described histologic reactions similar to those observed in the cardiac lesions of rheumatic fever. Similar results were obtained by other observers using a variety of antigens (Hawn and Janeway, 1947; More et al., 1949). Although "the morphologic equivalent" of rheumatic lesions was induced by these workers, none of them succeeded in demonstrating typical Aschoff bodies, the pathologic hallmark of rheumatic fever.

The Shwartzman reaction has also been used as an experimental model for the development of rheumatic lesions in animals. Myocardial necrosis was observed by Thomas et al. (1953) in rabbits by producing skin infections with group A streptococci followed by the intravenous injections of heterologous bacterial endotoxins. In this experimental model, lesions simulating rheumatic fever occurred without the development of an antigen-antibody reaction. Again, however, typical Aschoff bodies did not occur. Most observers agree that the changes noted in allergic reactions and in the Shwartzman phenomenon represent responses to tissue injury which are general in nature and not specific for rheumatic fever.

Group A streptococci are essentially human pathogens and only rarely cause spontaneous infections in animals. A number of attempts have been made to produce rheumatic fever by inoculating these organisms into animals by various routes. Watson et al. (1946) inoculated these organisms intranasally into monkeys but failed to induce cardiac lesions. Glaser et al. (1952) inoculated the pharyngeal tissues of rabbits with group A streptococci and succeeded in producing myocardial changes which resembled the lesions of rheumatic fever. The most extensive studies of group A streptococcal infections in animals have been reported by Murphy (1960). This author simulated the conditions as they occur in man by causing successive focal infections with group A streptococci of different types in rabbits. By comparing minutely the rabbit lesions with human rheumatic cardiac lesions obtained at autopsy or from left auricular appendages obtained at mitral commissurotomy, this observer has shown the close similarity of the cellular reactions observed in the rabbit and human tissues. These studies have led Murphy to believe that the Aschoff bodies are derived from myocardial fibers and not from connective tissue. The technique devised by Murphy has provided the best animal model available for the study of the cellular reactions similar to those caused by rheumatic fever and may yet prove a useful tool to shed light on the pathogenesis of this baffling disease.

Chapter Five

PATHOLOGY

The basic pathologic changes in rheumatic fever consist of exudative and proliferative inflammatory reactions in the mesenchymal supporting tissue of the heart, joints, blood vessels, and subcutaneous tissues. Lesions occur also in the pleura, lungs, and kidney, but are less common. The intensity of the exudative and proliferative processes varies with the site of involvement and the stage of the disease.

Initially there is edema of the ground substance, fragmentation of the collagen fibers, and a cellular infiltration of lymphocytes, plasma cells, and a few polymorphonuclear leukocytes. Scattered throughout the ground substance are deposits of an eosinophilic granular material termed fibrinoid. Early investigators believed that fibrinoid was derived from fragmented collagen fibers and rheumatic fever was classified therefore as one of the collagen diseases. However, the origin of fibrinoid has not been fully established. At present it is not considered to be a single substance but rather a complex material consisting of fibrin, gamma globulin, and other constituents (Gitlin et al., 1957; Vazquez and Dixon, 1958; Wagner, 1960). Fibrinoid changes occur in all connective tissue diseases, hypersensitivity states, and other conditions. Its appearance is probably a nonspecific response to tissue injury and it is unwarranted, therefore, to conclude that rheumatic fever is pathogenetically related to other conditions in which fibrinoid material is found.

THE ASCHOFF BODY

The distinctive pathognomonic lesion of rheumatic fever is the Aschoff body, first described by Aschoff in 1904. The Aschoff body is usually oval

33

in shape. It consists of a perivascular aggregation of large cells with polymorphous nuclei and basophilic cytoplasm arranged as a rosette around an avascular core of fibrinoid or necrotic protoplasm. Aschoff considered the Aschoff body as a specific lesion of the connective tissue and this view was generally accepted for 40 years.

This traditional concept has been challenged by Murphy (1960). On the basis of studies of cardiac tissues of 125 autopsies of patients dying of rheumatic fever and of 300 specimens of the left auricular appendage obtained at operation, this investigator believes that the Aschoff body is the result of injury to cardiac muscle fibers and that the connective tissue changes are secondary. Most pathologists disagree with Murphy's interpretation of his findings. The Aschoff cells differ in appearance from multinucleated cells known to arise from muscle; cross striations are not seen in transitional forms (Sokoloff, 1961). Histochemical studies of Aschoff cells suggest a closer relationship to connective tissue cells than to muscle fibers (Wagner, 1960). Furthermore Aschoff bodies have been observed in extracardiac lesions (Von Glahn, 1947). In a preliminary report based on electron microscopic studies, Lannigan and Zaki (1963) reported observations indicating that the Aschoff body did indeed originate from connective tissue. These investigators found no support for the view that this granuloma was derived from cardiac or smooth muscle.

A new and entirely different origin for the Aschoff body was suggested by Wedum and McGuire (1963). These workers published data suggesting that the Aschoff body is derived neither from connective tissue nor from cardiac muscle, but is formed as a result of blockage of the lymphatic channels of the heart. According to Wedum and McGuire, the rheumatic agent causes a proliferation of the endothelial cells lining the lymphatic vessels, and lymphatic drainage is thereby impaired. The Aschoff body is the result of injury to the lymphatic channel. The lack of adequate lymphatic drainage disturbs the metabolism of the cardiac musculature so that it no longer functions efficiently, and heart failure may result. These observations need confirmation.

Significance of the Aschoff Body

For many years pathologists have considered the Aschoff body an indication of an active rheumatic process. However, because of the high incidence of Aschoff bodies in biopsies of the left auricular appendage obtained at mitral commissurotomy from patients without clinical or laboratory signs of rheumatic activity, this concept is being re-examined. A number of observers have studied the correlation of Aschoff bodies in the biopsy specimens with morphologic evidence of rheumatic activity in other parts of the heart (Sabiston and Follis, 1952; Thomas et al., 1953; Decker et al., 1953; Kuschner and Levieff, 1953).

Kuschner and Levieff (1953), in a study of 40 necropsies, considered the following criteria indicative of an active process: (1) subendocardial or myocardial Aschoff bodies, (2) verrucous endocarditis of the valves, (3) the characteristic auriculitis of the posterior wall of the left atrium. In 9 of 40 specimens of the left auricular appendage, subendocardial Aschoff bodies were present, and in every instance active lesions were demonstrable in other parts of the heart. In 6, the auricular appendage was negative, although Aschoff bodies were found in the myocardium. In the remaining 25 cases both the auricular appendage and the remainder of the heart were negative for Aschoff bodies. These investigators concluded that when Aschoff bodies were present in the left auricular appendage, active rheumatic lesions were also present in other parts of the heart.

Most of the patients selected for mitral commissurotomy have no clinical signs of rheumatic activity, and in most instances the laboratory findings are also normal. Occasionally, however, the operation is performed despite an elevated sedimentation rate. Sabiston and Follis (1952) reported a higher incidence of Aschoff bodies in individuals with an increased sedimentation rate: in 32 patients undergoing mitral commissurotomy the ESR was elevated in 9 and normal in 23. The specimens obtained from the 9 patients with elevated sedimentation rates all showed Aschoff bodies, whereas in only 11 of the 23 patients with normal ESR's were Aschoff bodies found.

In an attempt to clarify the significance of Aschoff bodies found in biopsy specimens obtained from patients without signs of rheumatic activity, Tedeschi et al. (1955) classified Aschoff bodies as "active" or "senescent." "Active" Aschoff bodies showed an inflammatory reaction, or altered collagen or ground substance. "Senescent" Aschoff bodies were characterized by collagen hyalinization, scarring, or fibrosis. In a study of 400 biopsies only 8 (2 per cent) showed "active" Aschoff bodies. None of these 8 patients had signs of rheumatic activity, and no recrudescences of rheumatic fever occurred postoperatively. Sixty-seven (16.8 per cent) of the 400 specimens showed "senescent" Aschoff bodies. According to these investigators "senescent" Aschoff antibodies represent healing and are not indicative of an active rheumatic process.

Lannigan (1959) believes that the classification of Aschoff bodies as "active" or "senescent" is arbitrary. This investigator studied 175 biopsy specimens and found Aschoff bodies in 122 (64 per cent). Since half the patients studied had no history of rheumatic fever, Lannigan suggested that rheumatic carditis is mainly subclinical.

In older follow-up studies (Bland and Jones, 1951) the insidious development of valvular disease, especially mitral stenosis, was reported. In the opinion of Feinstein et al. (1964) rheumatic heart disease does not develop de novo. These observers believe that individuals who, after a period of years, are found to have organic heart disease are patients who had carditis without joint involvement or chorea. Because the characteristic overt symptoms of rheumatic fever were lacking, medical attention was not obtained at the time of the initial attack.

In more recent surveys, the appearance of delayed valvular heart disease is less common than formerly. Nevertheless occasionally some patients maintained on continuous prophylaxis and examined at regular intervals develop evidence of organic heart disease after varying lengths of time.

The frequent occurrence of Aschoff bodies in biopsies obtained at mitral commissurotomy from patients who have had no clinical or laboratory signs of rheumatic activity for many years has been observed repeatedly. It is now well established that when Aschoff bodies are present in the left auricular appendage, definite pathologic evidence of an active rheumatic process is usually demonstrable in other cardiac tissues. It is, therefore, impossible to be sure in any given individual precisely when cardiac involvement subsides completely. Apparently the inflammatory reaction is below the level necessary to produce clinical or laboratory abnormalities. Nevertheless it seems possible that the rheumatic agent which produces persistent and significant pathologic lesions may in some instances cause progressive cardiac damage.

An alternate explanation has been proposed by Magarey (1951) who suggested that organization of fibrin deposits on the valves may be of importance in the pathogenesis of chronic valvular disease. At the present time the significance of the Aschoff body is still not clear. However, the correlation of Aschoff bodies in the auricular appendage with active lesions in other cardiac tissues suggests that the rheumatic inflammatory process can occasionally persist late in the attack and that this process cannot be detected by current diagnostic tests.

PANCARDITIS

The rheumatic inflammatory process may involve all segments of the heart. Involvement of the heart muscle, *myocarditis*, is of paramount importance. During the acute stage there is often only a sparse inflammatory infiltration. However, cardiac dilatation and functional impairment of the heart may occur if the myocarditis is severe. As the disease progresses, Aschoff bodies appear in all portions of the myocardium but particularly in the subendocardial regions of the left ventricle and in the interventricular septum. After a variable period of time, the Aschoff cells assume the appearance of spindle-shaped fibrocytes and ultimately the site of the Aschoff body becomes a healed scar in the vicinity of blood vessels or lying between muscle bundles. There may be extensive fibrosis of the myocardium which can interfere with cardiac function and lead to hypertrophy of the heart.

Rheumatic *endocarditis* affects the mural endocardium and the valves. The most characteristic mural lesion is seen in the left atrium (MacCallum's patch) and is often visible grossly as a thickened opaque roughened area. The valvular lesion consists of edema and an inflammatory cellular reaction involving the leaflets and the chordae tendineae. Warty vegetations or verrucae appear along the line of closure. Microscopically the verrucae consist of hyaline masses. As the valvular lesions heal, the leaflets become thickened and deformed. The chordae tendineae shorten. The valve leaflets may fuse or they may curl and retract. After many years calcification of the scarred lesion may occur.

The valves of the left side of the heart are more frequently involved than those of the right. Disease of the mitral valve is the most common and frequently leads to mitral regurgitation. Mitral stenosis generally requires several years to develop. The aortic valve is the next most commonly affected either alone or in combination with mitral involvement. Aortic valvular disease may cause significant regurgitation early in the course of the disease. On the other hand, stenosis of the aortic valve takes many years to develop and is rarely encountered in childhood. The tricuspid valve is affected in a small percentage of patients and the pulmonic valve is rarely involved. The hemodynamic effects of valvular disease may lead ultimately to cardiac hypertrophy and dilatation.

Rheumatic *pericarditis* is common. Both the parietal and visceral layers are affected. The serous surfaces are red and roughened, and a fibrinous exudate occurs. The amount of fluid which accumulates varies greatly but is rarely large. The fluid is often turbid but never purulent. In long-standing cases the pericardium may become covered with a shaggy exudate which leads to adhesions between the visceral and parietal layers.

EXTRACARDIAC LESIONS

The inflammatory process in the *joints* is chiefly exudative and a variable amount of fluid collects in the joint space. Fibrinoid degeneration of the synovium may occur but the cartilage usually shows no change. The periarticular tissues are edematous and on occasion lesions similar to Aschoff bodies may be found. Histologically *subcutaneous nodules* contain a central area of fibrinoid necrotic material surrounded by connective tissue cells and varying numbers of lymphocytes. Their structure resembles that of the Aschoff body. They heal by proliferation of fibroblasts. Lesions of the *blood vessels* are commonly present and may be found anywhere in the body. The smaller vessels are involved chiefly, with swelling and proliferation of the endothelial cells which encroach upon the lumen. Fibrinous exudation and, at times, hemorrhage into the intima occurs.

Pathologic changes may be found in the *central nervous system*. Perivascular round cell infiltration, petechial hemorrhages, and hyalinization of small blood vessels have been reported in patients dying with chorea (Buchanan, 1941). Cellular changes scattered throughout the cortex, cerebellum, and basal ganglia have been described (Kernohan et al., 1939).

No site is consistently involved and Aschoff bodies have never been found in the brain. It has not been possible to correlate the clinical findings in chorea with pathologic changes in the central nervous system. Moreover, these changes have also been reported in patients with acute rheumatic fever who do not have chorea (Winkelman and Eckel, 1929).

The lungs may be involved although there is some question whether the pulmonary lesion is a rheumatic manifestation or a complication of heart failure. Rich and Gregory (1943) believe that the pulmonary lesion is the result of focal damage to the small blood vessels, particularly the alveolar capillaries. In the most recent report, Goldring et al. (1958) described the pulmonary findings in 16 patients in whom a diagnosis of "rheumatic pneumonia" was made. Grossly the lungs had a hemorrhagic appearance. Fibrin and hemosiderin deposits in the alveoli were common. Fifty per cent of the patients had hyaline membrane formation. There was evidence of a bacterial pneumonia in less than half of the patients. Aschoff bodies have never been found in the lungs. It is the opinion of most observers that the pathologic changes are not specific for rheumatic fever.

Rheumatic *serositis* may occur. As has already been noted, involvement of pericardium is not uncommon but it is virtually never found in the absence of lesions in the myocardium and endocardium. A serous or serofibrinous exudate of the pleura may occur. Peritoneal involvement is less common and the findings are usually minimal. In rheumatic subjects with abdominal pain who have been operated upon for suspected appendicitis, a small amount of free fluid may be found. The peritoneum may appear slightly edematous but it not infrequently appears grossly normal.

Chapter Six

CLINICAL MANIFESTATIONS
OF ACUTE RHEUMATIC
FEVER

INTRODUCTION

The signs and symptoms of acute rheumatic fever vary greatly. The clinical findings are determined by the sites of involvement, the severity of the lesions, the time of appearance during the course of the illness, and the stage at which the patient is first examined. Certain of the clinical findings are found with such frequency in this disease as to make them diagnostically important. They have been designated the *major manifestations* and include carditis, arthritis, chorea, subcutaneous nodules, and erythema marginatum. The term "major" does not relate to severity or to the activity of rheumatic process and has no prognostic significance.

In addition to the five chief manifestations, there are a number of other signs and symptoms which are frequently associated with rheumatic fever. Some, such as fever and arthralgia, although not pathognomonic for rheumatic fever, may be helpful in establishing the diagnosis and are classified as *minor manifestations*. Epistaxis, abdominal pain, and rheumatic pneumonia are additional features that may be part of the clinical syndrome but rarely aid in the diagnosis. The clinical findings associated with each of these manifestations are described in this section. Problems related to diagnosis are mentioned only briefly since they are discussed more fully in a separate chapter.

CARDITIS

The term rheumatic carditis indicates an active inflammatory process involving the myocardium, endocardium, or pericardium, usually in combination. *Carditis is the most important of the major rheumatic manifestations for it is the only one which results in sequelae.* In its most fulminant form it can cause death in the acute stage of the disease. Fortunately this severe type of carditis has become rare and at present occurs in less than 1 per cent of the patients. More often the inflammatory process in the myocardium is less intense and the predominant lesion is in the heart valves. Complete healing may occur, or permanent valvular deformities and chronic rheumatic heart disease may follow. Permanent valvular lesions are more likely to develop in children with severe carditis. During their first attack, however, even patients with cardiac decompensation may recover completely. Rheumatic heart disease also occurs in children in whom no history of a rheumatic episode is obtainable. Between these two extremes, there are many variations in the mode of onset, the association with other rheumatic manifestations, the severity of the cardiac involvement, and the ultimate outcome.

Incidence

The incidence of carditis in initial attacks of rheumatic fever reported by different observers during a 12 year period (1951 to 1963) varies from 40 to 51 per cent (Table 6). In a series of 168 children with acute rheumatic fever seen between 1959 and 1963, unequivocal clinical evidence of carditis was found in 40 per cent (Combined Rheumatic Fever Study Group, 1965). The frequency of carditis appears to be decreasing. Sixty-five per cent of the children with acute rheumatic fever admitted to the Bellevue Hospital between 1935 and 1942 had carditis as compared with 44 per cent between 1951 and 1958 (Mayer et al., 1963). In a 40 year study from The House of the Good Samaritan, cardiac involvement occurred in 73 per cent of the children admitted between 1921 and 1930 and declined to 51 per cent during 1951 to 1960 (Massell et al., 1964).

Clinical Patterns of Carditis

The clinical picture associated with rheumatic carditis and the time at which the cardiac findings appear are variable. However, several clinical patterns occur with some regularity.

The acute rheumatic attack in children over 6 years of age is heralded most frequently by fever and arthritis, complaints which bring the patient to medical attention. In these children there are often no symptoms referable to heart unless pericarditis is present. The physical signs of carditis

Table 6. Incidence of Carditis among Children with First Attacks
of Acute Rheumatic Fever

Authors	Period	No. Patients	% with Carditis
Combined Rheumatic Fever Study Group (1960, 1965)	1959-1963	168	40
Feinstein et al. (1962)	1958-1960	275	42
Mayer et al. (1963)	1951-1958	200	44
Massell et al. (1964)	1951-1960	1125	51

in many children may be noted at the time of the first examination. However, at times the cardiac findings are normal or equivocal at the onset,
and become abnormal over the course of several days or, at the most,
within one to two weeks. Massell and co-workers (1958) have pointed
out that patients with an acute onset of rheumatic fever rarely show a *long*
delay in the appearance of carditis if this manifestation is going to occur.
In their large series of patients, 76 per cent of the patients with evidence
of heart damage had cardiac involvement during the first week of illness.

A second and not uncommon pattern of childhood rheumatic fever
associated with carditis begins much more insidiously. There may be a
history of a slight fever and joint pains over a period of several weeks.
Frequently the symptoms are vague and not at all distinctive. The child
loses his appetite, appears sallow, and tires more easily. The presenting
complaint may be shortness of breath or chest pain. These children appear
subacutely or chronically ill. There is often a striking degree of facial
pallor. A low-grade fever and vague joint tenderness may be present at
the time of the initial examination, but in general the clinical evidence of
an inflammatory state is usually minimal. In contrast, the signs of cardiac
involvement are unequivocal and not infrequently even include evidence
of early congestive heart failure. The incidence and severity of carditis
appears to be greater in children who have an insidious onset as compared to patients who manifest high fever and severe arthritis at the beginning of an attack. It is possible that in the latter group carditis is generally
milder because treatment is instituted earlier. However, this explanation
has been questioned by some observers (Feinstein and Spagnuolo, 1962).

The presence of active rheumatic carditis may be recognized for the
first time in children whose presenting complaint is chorea. There is usually no history of joint symptoms. They are afebrile and evidence of inflammation may be limited to an elevated sedimentation rate. The cardiac signs
are often the only findings which distinguish these children from the
group with so-called "pure" chorea.

Signs of Carditis

The clinical signs associated with rheumatic carditis vary with the nature and the degree of cardiac involvement. There are four well known signs: (1) significant murmurs not previously present, (2) enlargement of the heart, (3) cardiac decompensation, and (4) a pericardial friction rub or effusion. If either one or more of these findings are unequivocally present in a patient with active rheumatic fever, the diagnosis of carditis is justified.

Murmurs. Rheumatic carditis is almost always associated with a significant murmur. Auscultation should be performed with great care, therefore, and at repeated intervals in every patient suspected of rheumatic fever. The diagnosis of carditis must always be considered in doubt if a significant murmur is not heard at any time during the course of the illness. There are two exceptions. A murmur may be obscured or absent in patients with a pericardial rub or marked effusion. In addition in the early stages of rheumatic fever, particularly in children less than 6 years of age, there may be evidence of myocarditis with enlargement and even signs of congestive heart failure without significant murmurs.

The mitral valve is the most common valvular site of rheumatic inflammation and it is involved three times more frequently than the aortic valve. Mitral valvulitis may lead to mitral regurgitation early in the course of the illness. The characteristic auscultatory finding is a systolic murmur heard maximally at the apex, blowing and high-pitched in quality, filling all of systole and transmitted toward the axilla. The loudness of the murmur varies between grades 2 and 4 (on a scale of 6). It may change in intensity early in the course of the illness. Initially it may be very soft. The intensity depends not only on the degree of regurgitation but on the state of myocardial function, the thickness of the chest wall, and other factors. For these reasons loudness alone may be misleading, and the other characteristics mentioned, particularly the quality and the duration of the murmur, must be taken into consideration. It is important to distinguish the significant systolic murmur from the innocent bruits heard so commonly in children. The characteristics of the innocent or functional murmurs of childhood are described more fully in the chapter on diagnosis (page 87).

In a considerable proportion of patients with mitral valvulitis, the systolic murmur is accompanied by a mid-diastolic murmur (Carey-Coombs murmur). This murmur begins directly after the onset of the third heart sound. It may be due either to vibrations set up by the abrupt stretching of the heart muscle (Luisada et al., 1955) or to a sudden increase in the tautness of the mitral cusps and chordae (Nixon, 1961). It is low-pitched, has a variable duration, and is localized to a small area at or just above the apex. It is heard best with the bell portion of the stethoscope pressed lightly against the chest wall with the patient in the left lateral position. It is often transient and may easily be missed. Identification of the mid-diastolic murmur is of importance in acute rheumatic fever, because it occurs only if there is definite mitral valvulitis and its presence confirms the significance of the apical systolic murmur. The mid-diastolic murmur may be easily confused with a third heart sound. The latter occurs frequently in acute rheumatic carditis, but it is also found commonly in normal children or during febrile states due to other causes. The mid-diastolic murmur of acute valvulitis should not be mistaken for the murmur of mitral stenosis which takes months or years to develop. The murmur of mitral stenosis is longer and has a presystolic accentuation; when there is doubt about the presystolic quality, exercise often will bring out its special characteristics.

It has already been noted that the aortic valve is less commonly involved than the mitral. When aortic valvulitis does occur, the basal diastolic murmur of aortic regurgitation may appear early in the course of the disease. At times its appearance is quite sudden. Its presence always indicates significant carditis and it is of considerable diagnostic and prognostic importance. It may occur alone or with mitral valvulitis. At the onset, this murmur is soft and is heard very early in diastole after the second sound. It may be audible only intermittently. It is usually loudest at the third interspace at the left border of the sternum, but at times it is heard best at the second interspace to the right of the sternum. It varies in intensity and pitch and may be difficult to detect (Feinstein and DiMassa, 1959). It is heard best with the diaphragm portion of the stethoscope and sometimes can be detected when the patient leans forward and holds his breath in expiration. As the regurgitant flow increases, the diastolic murmur becomes louder and acquires a more characteristic high-pitched decrescendo quality. Widening of the pulse pressure is rarely an early finding.

Basal systolic murmurs are sometimes heard in children with acute rheumatic carditis. They may be due to an anterior, upward radiation of a loud apical systolic murmur. Usually, however, they can be heard separately from the murmur of mitral regurgitation. They have a short ejection quality and are probably physiologic sounds associated with the flow of blood from the left ventricle into the great vessels. Basal systolic murmurs are not the result of rheumatic aortic stenosis, a lesion that is uncommon in childhood and only occurs years after the acute attack.

Cardiac Enlargement. Dilatation of the cardiac chambers, particularly the left ventricle, is a common finding in acute rheumatic carditis. Cardiomegaly occurred in 53.8 per cent of children with carditis in two carefully documented studies (Combined Rheumatic Fever Study Group, 1960, 1965). The detection of enlargement is of considerable importance since it may confirm the diagnosis of carditis in doubtful cases. Moreover, cardiomegaly means that there has been significant involvement of the myocardium by the acute inflammatory process. The degree of enlargement, therefore, is a valuable index of severity and it is a useful parameter in observing the course of the patient.

Careful attention must be paid to localization of the apical impulse. A diffuse impulse should always suggest dilation of the heart. When cardiomegaly is more pronounced, the apical impulse is displaced downward and to the left and percussion of the left border will reveal dullness beyond the midclavicular line. If pericardial effusion is present, there may be dullness beyond the apical impulse. It is usually difficult to detect mild enlargement on physical examination. A more accurate determination can be obtained by chest x-ray. The radiographic findings are discussed separately (Chapter 8).

Congestive Heart Failure. In keeping with the declining severity of rheumatic fever, heart failure is seen less commonly at the present time. It is not rare, however, and still occurs in 5 to 10 per cent of first attacks of rheumatic carditis. It is more frequent in children under 6 years of age. As has already been noted, the child who has been ill with low-grade fever and arthralgia for several weeks is more likely to present with symptoms and signs of cardiac decompensation than the patient with an abrupt onset of fever and polyarthritis. Congestive heart failure is more common in children with recurrent attacks.

Cough, chest pain, shortness of breath, marked fatigue, sweating, and anorexia are symptoms of heart failure. Palpitations and upper abdominal pain are less common complaints in children than in adults. Indeed, some children have remarkably few symptoms even though signs of decompensation are present on examination. The physical findings are variable and depend on the degree and duration of the heart failure. In the pediatric age group, particularly in young children, it is often difficult to make a sharp distinction between right-sided and left-sided heart failure. The signs in patients with an initial attack of carditis may be minimal, limited only to an increase in respiratory rate. Hepatomegaly is a common and valuable sign of decompensation and should be sought for assiduously. At times it may be difficult to palpate the liver; tenderness over the hepatic region may be a clue to engorgement of the liver. A protodiastolic gallop occurs commonly and should alert the physician to the possibility of impending failure. The pulmonary findings are most variable. The clinical picture of acute pulmonary edema with frothy sputum and wet lung fields is seen only in the fulminant form of acute myocarditis which is rare at the present time. More often the clinical signs of congestion of the lungs are either entirely absent or limited to a few basilar rales, even though heart failure is suspected on the basis of dyspnea or the presence of vascular congestion on the x-ray. At times, the chest roentgenogram may yield the only clue that incipient heart failure is indeed present. Edema of the dependent parts is usually present only in patients who have been ambulatory for some time. Puffiness about the face is more common in children than pitting edema. Distention of the neck veins may be present but it is neither an early nor a common finding.

Signs of cardiac decompensation may occur during the course of any attack of active rheumatic carditis and patients should be examined frequently and carefully for this complication. Tachypnea associated with salicylism and enlarged liver secondary to steroid therapy should not be mistaken for signs of heart failure.

It is axiomatic that the presence of heart failure in children with a recent attack of rheumatic fever denotes active carditis. However in patients with a known previous attack of rheumatic fever it is often difficult to know on the basis of the clinical findings if the onset of heart failure is due to a recurrence of rheumatic fever or to a complication of long-standing valvular disease. The presence of other rheumatic manifestations or evidence of a recent streptococcal infection favor the diagnosis of a recurrence.

Pericarditis. The pericardium may be involved in the acute inflammatory rheumatic process. It is perhaps the least common of the important clinical findings in acute carditis. Pericarditis was noted in 38 of 497 children in one study (U.K. and U.S. Joint Report, 1955) and in essentially the same number (29 of 457) in another large series (Massell et al., 1958). It occurs in the severe forms of rheumatic carditis as a component of pancarditis. Although it is rarely an isolated finding, there are occasions when the pericardium appears to be affected to a much greater degree than the myocardium or endocardium. In such patients the cardiac findings may regress rapidly following antirheumatic treatment and the course of the illness may be quite benign. Involvement of the pericardium subsides without clinical residua.

Pericarditis should always be suspected in children with acute rheumatic fever and chest pain. Indeed, chest pain and fever may be the only presenting complaints in some patients. More often pericarditis is discovered only after a friction rub has been heard during the physical examination. This may be present at the onset or appear during the course of an attack. It is always a sign of active disease. The friction rub is one of the most characteristic signs in clinical medicine and it is pathognomonic for pericarditis. The rub is a superficial scratching or grating sound heard loudest at the base and along the left sternal border. It may be evanescent. At times it is widely distributed over the precordium or it may be localized near the apex. It is heard usually in both phases of the cardiac cycle. However it may be audible only during systole or diastole, especially early in the course of the illness, and it may occasionally be confused with a high-pitched systolic murmur or the diastolic murmur of aortic insufficiency. Pericarditis is often associated with other auscultatory evidence of rheumatic carditis. However, a loud rub may obscure cardiac murmurs and a clinical assessment of the endocardial involvement may have to be deferred.

Effusion is additional evidence of pericarditis. It should be suspected if there is a marked widening of percussion dullness of the cardiac borders or if both heart sounds are unusually muffled. The effusion caused by rheumatic pericarditis is rarely large and for that reason many of the clinical signs usually associated with effusion may be absent. Often it can be recognized only in the chest roentgenogram and even then it may be difficult to distinguish effusion from cardiac dilatation. The radiographic findings are discussed elsewhere (page 71). The electrocardiographic abnormalities of pericarditis are also discussed in a separate section (page 79).

Other Cardiac Findings

In addition to the four chief signs of carditis outlined above, there are often other clinical cardiac findings such as tachycardia, changes in heart sounds, a gallop rhythm, and arrhythmias. When the latter signs occur in patients with acute rheumatic fever, the diagnosis of carditis may be suspected but not considered a certainty unless one or more of the four diagnostic signs appear.

Tachycardia. A rapid pulse rate is an important finding if it is disproportionate to the fever. It can be evaluated properly only when fever has been reduced. Common causes of tachycardia in children are apprehension and excitement. It is therefore advisable to keep a careful hospital record of the sleeping pulse in every child with acute or suspected rheumatic fever. A sleeping pulse of over 100 is a bona fide sign of carditis. A sinus bradycardia of less than 60 beats per minute is occasionally seen in patients with acute carditis.

Heart Sounds. Both the first and the second heart sounds may be distant if significant effusion is present. A more common event in acute rheumatic fever is the diminution in the intensity of the first heart sounds. This finding can serve as a clinical clue to the presence of first degree heart block. With a delay in atrioventricular conduction, the ventricles contract at a longer time than normal after the atria, allowing the mitral leaflets to float back up to a higher position. When ventricular systole does occur, the sound produced by the closing mitral valve is faint. Variations in intensity of the first sound should suggest a changing PR interval. These changes may be associated with progressive lengthening of the PR interval, the so-called Wenckebach phenomenon. A diminished first heart sound and prolonged atrioventricular conduction time are not by themselves significant signs of carditis. When they are isolated findings, it is rare for the patient to develop valvular disease later.

Gallop Rhythm. A protodiastolic gallop rhythm is often noted with congestive heart failure and its occurrence may herald the onset of decompensation. On the other hand, a gallop rhythm may be heard in children with a prominent physiologic third heart sound and a tachycardia due to any cause. This finding should not be overinterpreted, therefore, in patients without other evidence of carditis.

Arrhythmias. Changes in cardiac rhythm may occur during acute rheumatic carditis. Premature beats and arrhythmias associated with heart block and interference dissociation can occur. Atrial fibrillation is rarely caused by acute rheumatic fever but is not uncommon in patients with long-standing mitral valvular disease.

Diagnosis

The occurrence of a newly acquired organic heart murmur, cardiac enlargement, pericarditis, or congestive heart failure in a patient with acute rheumatic fever makes the diagnosis of carditis self-evident. Not infrequently, however, patients with acute rheumatic fever have equivocal cardiac findings which may or may not be transient, and must be carefully evaluated. In other instances, the diagnosis of rheumatic fever is doubtful, and the signs indicative of carditis may be of viral origin or due to other nonrheumatic causes. The differential diagnosis is discussed in Chapter 9.

JOINT MANIFESTATIONS

Arthritis

Joint symptoms are the most common presenting complaint in rheumatic fever in children over six years of age. Arthritis, a *major manifestation* of this disease, occurs in about three-quarters of patients during the acute stage of rheumatic fever. In earlier reports the incidence of this manifestation ranged between 62 and 85 per cent (Coombs, 1924; Coburn, 1931). The frequency has not changed over the years.

Clinical Findings. The symptoms and signs referable to the joints vary markedly. Usually the larger joints are involved, particularly the knees, ankles, elbows, and wrists. In general the hips are less commonly affected and the spine is almost never involved. The small joints of the fingers and toes are not commonly affected. Several joints may be involved simultaneously or, more characteristically, the inflammatory process migrates from joint to joint over a period of several days. Occasionally the findings are limited to one joint, but frequently in such a patient either a history of tenderness in other joints can be elicited on careful questioning or additional joints become involved within a few days if antirheumatic agents are withheld.

In rheumatic fever more than any other joint disease, the pain is often disproportionate to the objective joint findings. Not infrequently it is so exquisite that the slightest pressure causes excruciating pain. It may be localized to one area over the joint but it is more often diffuse, radiates to the periarticular tissues, and on occasion causes spasm of the surrounding muscles. Local heat, redness, and swelling may be present. The redness is often limited to a small area over the involved joint. If there is swelling, it is diffuse and nonpitting, and not otherwise characteristic.

The duration of involvement of each joint in untreated patients varies from 1 to 5 days, rarely longer. The joint symptoms usually subside in 2 to 4 weeks even without treatment. Exacerbations may occur within a 1 to 2 week period after antirheumatic agents are discontinued. In contrast to rheumatoid arthritis, rheumatic fever never causes permanent deformities to the joints.*

Joint involvement rarely occurs simultaneously with active chorea. However, chorea may follow the arthritis; only rarely is the reverse true. The incidence and severity of cardiac involvement appears to be lower in patients with severe polyarthritis than in those with milder joint manifestations. Feinstein and Spagnuolo (1962) observed carditis in 26 per cent of patients with red, hot, or swollen joints, in 40 per cent of those with tender joints, and in 96 per cent of children with arthralgia (Table 7). Our own observations on the relationship of the severity of the joint involvement to the incidence of carditis among 129 patients studied since 1959 are essentially in accord with those of these investigators. It is not clear why patients with severe joint involvement tend to have less heart disease. However it is clinically useful to know that the prognosis in patients with red, hot, swollen joints is generally better than in children with a less abrupt onset.

Arthralgia

Pain around the joints without any objective findings is a common complaint in active rheumatic fever. In the absence of overt arthritis, arthralgia is considered a *minor manifestation*. The joint manifestations may be limited entirely to arthralgia during the entire course of an acute attack. It may precede or follow other rheumatic manifestations, recurring over a period of days or several weeks. Definite arthritis may be present in a single joint or in several joints and only arthralgia in others.

Clinical Findings. The symptoms occur intermittently and vary in severity. Occasionally the pain may be severe enough to incapacitate the child, or cause a slight limp or only very mild complaints. The pain may be aggravated by exercise and at times may simulate injury to a joint. It is usually worse during the day and is not relieved by heat or local applications. The larger joints are usually involved, often in a migratory

* Bywaters (1950) has reported an instance of the so-called Jaccoud type of chronic rheumatism affecting the metacarpophalangeal joints in a patient with rheumatic fever. This condition is due to periarticular fibrosis rather than synovitis. The etiology and its relationship to rheumatic fever are not known.

Table 7. Severity of Joint Symptoms and Cardiac Involvement*

Severity of Joint Symptoms	Number of Patients	Number and Per Cent of Patients with Carditis
Red, hot, or swollen joints	179	47 (26%)
Tender joints	30	12 (40%)
Joint pains	25	24 (96%)
No joint symptoms	29	29 (100%)

* Modified from Feinstein and Spagnuolo: Medicine 41:279, 1962.

fashion. There is no redness, swelling, or heat. There may or may not be slight limitation of motion. Sometimes vague tenderness may be elicited by deep pressure. Since examination of the joints is often negative, questioning of the child as well as detailed history from the parent are needed to ascertain whether the pain is in the joint or merely muscular.

Diagnosis

The classic picture of the febrile child with heat, redness, and tenderness of first one joint and then another is a readily recognizable clinical syndrome of rheumatic fever. On the other hand, many of the diagnostic dilemmas in this disease stem from difficulties in evaluating mild and atypical arthritis or arthralgia. The differential diagnosis is discussed more fully in another chapter (page 85).

CHOREA

Chorea minor (Sydenham's chorea, St. Vitus' dance) is a disorder of the central nervous system characterized by emotional instability, purposeless movements, and muscular weakness. It is a major manifestation of rheumatic fever. Chorea occurs most commonly between the ages of 7 and 14 years, with the peak incidence at 8 years. It is more common in girls than in boys. It is rare after puberty and is exceedingly uncommon after the age of 20 years.

Incidence

In a series of 1000 cases of rheumatic fever published by Bland and Jones (1951), 518 patients, slightly more than half, had chorea. In an analysis of 362 initial attacks of rheumatic fever admitted to the pediatric service of Bellevue Hospital in New York City, 255 children had chorea (Mayer et al., 1963). In 73 of the 255 patients, arthritis or carditis was present in addition to chorea. In the remaining 182 children (70 per cent) chorea occurred without other signs of rheumatic fever ("pure" chorea). This study spanned 24 years from 1935 through 1958. Throughout this period the incidence of chorea accompanied by arthritis or carditis remained essentially the same. During the last 8 years, from 1951 through 1958, the number of children admitted with "pure" chorea showed a decrease of approximately 50 per cent. A similar trend was observed at The House of the Good Samaritan in Boston: from 1921 to 1925 43 per cent of the patients admitted had chorea as compared to 15 per cent of those admitted from 1956 to 1960 (Massell et al., 1964).

Relationship of "Pure" Chorea to Rheumatic Fever

Cheadle in 1889 was the first to include chorea as part of the rheumatic syndrome, and at the present time chorea is classified as one of the major manifestations of this disease. Chorea may occur alone or be accompanied by other rheumatic signs and symptoms. Because chorea may occur in the absence of other evidence of rheumatic inflammation, so-called "pure" chorea, some observers have doubted a rheumatic etiology (Gerstley et al., 1935; Coburn and Moore, 1937; Kagan and Mirman, 1947).

Patients with "pure" chorea differ markedly from patients with polyarthritis or carditis. They are afebrile, and clinical and laboratory signs indicative of rheumatic inflammation are absent. No history of a preceding upper respiratory infection is obtained and streptococcal antibodies may be within the normal range. However, in 1956, Taranta and Stollerman showed that chorea, like polyarthritis and carditis, is a complication of streptococcal pharyngitis. Chorea differs from polyarthritis and carditis in that the latent period between the upper respiratory infection and the appearance of chorea is much longer. Instead of the usual one to 3 weeks, it may vary from one to 6 months (Fig. 4). After this long interval streptococcal antibodies in many instances have returned to normal levels. Taranta (1959) followed 60 children with "pure" chorea in a special prophylactic clinic where throat cultures and streptococcal antibody determinations were obtained at frequent intervals. Nineteen of these 60 patients had streptococcal infections and 3 of these 19 children had recurrences of "pure" chorea 3 to 6 months after the first serologic evidence of the streptococcal infection. These data suggest that recurrences of "pure" chorea may occur at long intervals after the streptococcal infection and in the absence of other rheumatic manifestations.

Symptoms and signs of chorea have been reported in a number of different diseases such as systemic lupus erythematosus, Henoch-Schönlein syndrome and polycythemia vera. In the case of systemic lupus erythematosus reported by Paradise (1960) the patient had unequivocal serologic evidence of an intercurrent streptococcal infection. When chorea is observed during the course of other diseases it is essential to rule out intercurrent streptococcal infections by antibody studies. In general it is best to follow the advice of Poynton and Holmes (1913): "Chorea is

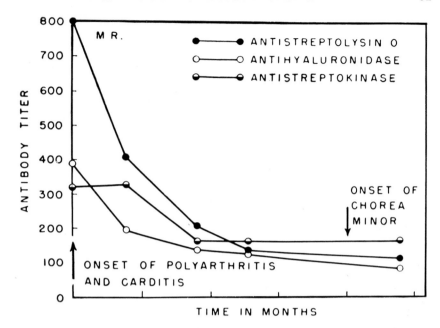

Figure 4. Chorea appearing 4 months after the onset of polyarthritis and carditis without evidence of an intercurrent infection. (From Taranta and Stollerman: Amer. J. Med. *20*:170, 1956.)

mostly rheumatic and . . . when chorea occurs without any history of rheumatism it is presumably the primary rheumatic symptom and in practical medicine is best looked on as a stamp of rheumatism."

Emotional Factors and Chorea

Emotional factors have been implicated in chorea since the time of Sydenham. There are some children with chorea in whom there is a history of an acute emotional stress prior to the onset of overt symptoms, but it seems possible that in these patients, choreic manifestations already present may have become more pronounced. Emotional lability and behavior disturbances are characteristic of the chorea syndrome. It has been suggested that chorea which is not associated with other rheumatic manifestations (so-called "pure" chorea) may have a different etiology, possibly psychogenic (Gerstley et al., 1935; Kagan and Mirman, 1947). However, as has been noted, the bulk of the evidence does not favor a separate etiology for "pure" chorea.

Chapman and co-workers (1958) carried out a psychosomatic study of 8 children with chorea and found that their personalities were abnormal and were characterized by marked passivity, much underlying anxiety, and schizoid withdrawal. Three of the children had a history of rheumatic fever and in two others the evidence was equivocal. The authors concluded that a personality disorder as well as rheumatic fever may be a factor in the pathogenesis of chorea. These findings differed from the results obtained by Sachs and co-workers (1962). They performed psychologic tests on 10 patients with acute chorea, on 10 who had recovered from chorea, and on matched controls who had rheumatic fever without chorea. They found no evidence that patients with chorea had abnormal personalities or that chorea per se created any significant psychologic disturbances. They suggested that the emotional difficulties which occurred during the course of an attack were related to the motor impairment.

Pregnancy and Chorea

During a 34 year period, 1910 to 1944, Lewis-Jonsson (1949) studied 477 women with chorea. In 17 of these 477 patients, choreic manifestations developed during pregnancy. Of the 17 patients, 13 were para I, 3 para II and one para V. Among 14 women for whom the trimester is recorded, chorea developed during the first trimester in 6, in 3 during the second, and in 5 during the third. Ten of the 17 women had had no previous attacks, 5 had had previous attacks. The interval between the first attack and the pregnancy varied from 6 to 16 years. In 2 it was not stated whether they had had previous atacks.

In this country chorea during pregnancy appears to be less common. Among 50,000 pregnant women, Eastman (1956) in Baltimore during a 20 year period observed a single mild case.

Pathophysiology

The histologic changes vary from case to case and are not localized to any area. It has not been possible to correlate these changes with the clinical symptoms and the neurologic findings. Buchanan et al. (1942) have suggested that there is a release of inhibitory mechanisms from extrapyramidal or cerebellar sources. Recent studies of the "H" reflex tend to support this hypothesis (Hodes et al., 1962). The "H" reflex is a monosynaptic stretch reflex elicited by percutaneous stimulation. It is normally suppressed by 6 months of age but in patients with chorea the "H" reflex can be elicited and it disappears as the chorea subsides.

Electroencephalographic abnormalities have been noted in patients with chorea (Usher and Jasper, 1941). Studies have demonstrated a diffuse dysrhythmia with slow activity of increased amplitude. Similar findings have been reported by Diamond and Tentler (1962). These observers found no brain wave abnormalities in rheumatic patients without chorea. The significance of the electroencephalographic abnormalities is not known.

Clinical Findings

Chorea may appear several weeks after an attack of acute rheumatic fever or it may be the initial symptom of a rheumatic episode. The onset is usually gradual. A child, previously well controlled, becomes increasingly nervous. He tends to drop things and stumbles frequently. Often the school teacher reports grimacing and writing difficulties. Speech becomes indistinct, and characteristic purposeless movements of the arms and the legs develop. The movements are increased by effort, excitement, and fatigue, but cease when the patient is asleep. Muscular weakness is common, and the child may be unable to walk, talk, or even sit up. Often the movements are so violent that the patient has to be placed in a padded crib to prevent injury. Infrequently only one side of the body is involved (hemichorea).

Certain clinical maneuvers may bring out signs of chorea. In mild cases, the movements can be exaggerated after periods of direct questioning or enforced quiet. Dysfunction of speech may be elicited by having the child count rapidly; for the first few numbers he may speak clearly, and then suddenly the speech becomes thick, or he hesitates or is unable to utter a sound for several seconds. When he talks, there may be a clucking sound, due to sudden contraction of the tongue to the floor of the mouth. There is only slight resistance to passive movements. The hand grasp is frequently weak and may consist of spasmodic contractions followed by rapid relaxation. Fibrillary twitchings of the muscles may also be detected while the hand is held. There may be a broad grin one moment, followed suddenly by a "poker face" or even a tearful expression. When the tongue is protruded, it is impossible to hold it quietly, and its undulating, jerky movements have been described as those of a bag of worms. The child may bite the tongue to keep it protruded. If he is asked to extend his arms with outstretched fingers in front of him, he soon hyperextends his wrists and fingers; or if he is asked to raise his arms above his head, he soon turns his arms so that the backs of the hands oppose. With deep breathing the diaphragm may be drawn upward so that the abdominal wall is drawn inward. The response to the patellar reflex is often "hung-up."

Other signs of rheumatic inflammation may be present and should be sought for carefully in every patient with chorea. Active carditis is found in a significant number of children whose initial complaint is chorea. The carditis is usually not severe and, indeed, the signs of cardiac involvement may be missed unless careful and repeated examinations of the heart are performed. Active arthritis rarely occurs concurrently with chorea.

Diagnosis

The diagnosis of chorea is usually unmistakable in the child with the fully developed clinical syndrome. The history of an insidious onset, the bizarre purposeless movements, the emotional changes, and muscle weakness are all characteristic. In the early stages of the illness, however, it may be exceedingly difficult to make the diagnosis. The differential diagnosis is discussed fully in Chapter 9, page 92.

Clinical Course and Prognosis

Chorea is a self-limited condition and there is usually complete recovery from the emotional and neuromuscular abnormalities. However, the course of the illness is extremely variable. Mild cases may subside within a few weeks. On the other hand, in some patients the emotional and motor changes increase slowly over a period of weeks and remain at a maximal level for several more weeks before they begin to subside. In the average case recovery usually occurs in 3 months. Relapses are not uncommon, and occasionally signs of chorea may wax and wane for a year or more.

The prognosis of patients with chorea *and* rheumatic fever does not differ from that of patients with rheumatic fever alone. However, in children with "pure" chorea, it is usually stated that the prognosis in terms of heart disease is generally good. This view was based chiefly on a report by Jones and Bland in 1935. These observers found that of 134 children with "pure" chorea followed for an average of 8 years, only 4 (3 per cent) had residual heart disease. Subsequently, Sutton and Dodge (1938) found that among 91 children with "pure" chorea followed for an average of 4.8 years, 17 (18.6 per cent) had heart disease. In a more recent study from Boston, Bland (1961) reported follow-up observations on patients with "pure" chorea originally reported by Jones and Bland (1935). During a 20 year period, the percentage of patients with rheu-

Table 8.   Delayed Appearance of Rheumatic Heart Disease after "Pure" Chorea: 163 Cases*

	At the Time of Chorea	Years after Onset			
		1-5	6-10	11-15	16-20
R. H. D.	6	3	10	10	9
Cumulative per cent	3.4	5.5	11.6	17.8	23.3

* From Bland, E. F.: Trans. Amer. Clin. Climat. Ass. 73:209, 1961.

matic heart disease increased progressively from 3 to 23.3 per cent (Table 8). Recurrences of chorea occurred frequently but no other rheumatic manifestations were recorded. From these data it would appear that "pure" chorea does not have a uniformly good prognosis. However, most of the patients did not have the benefit of prophylaxis. Although long-term studies on the effect of prophylaxis on the prognosis of patients with "pure" chorea are not available, on the basis of evidence presented by Taranta such individuals should receive continuous prophylaxis (Neimann, 1963).

Treatment

See the chapter on treatment, page 109.

SUBCUTANEOUS NODULES

Subcutaneous nodules are one of the most characteristic of the *major manifestations* of active rheumatic fever and occur most commonly in children with severe carditis of several weeks' duration.

Incidence

The incidence of this manifestation varies in different countries as well as in different parts of the United States. In a large series of patients from two continents, subcutaneous nodules were noted in 21.7 per cent of the United Kingdom patients as compared to 7.4 per cent of children with rheumatic fever from this country (U.K. and U.S. Joint Report, 1955). Nodules have been found in approximately 10 per cent of rheumatic children in Boston (Massell et al., 1958), but they occur in not more than 2 per cent of patients seen in Baltimore. The reasons for these unusual geographical variations are not clear. The incidence of nodules does not appear to have decreased, at least not in the environs of New York City. Baldwin and co-workers (1960) studied the frequency of nodules among children admitted to the Bellevue Hospital between 1928 and 1942 and 1953 and 1958 and found an incidence of approximately 10 per cent during both periods. In view of the declining severity of rheumatic fever, it is surprising that the incidence of nodules has not changed.

Clinical Findings

Nodules are almost never present in the early stages of acute rheumatic fever and they usually do not appear until several weeks after the onset of the attack. Their presence at the time of the initial examination signifies, therefore, that the rheumatic episode is not of recent onset.

Nodules are hard, painless, non-pruritic swellings which are freely movable. The skin overlying the nodule is not discolored. They are usually found over the extensor surfaces of the joints, notably the elbows, knuckles, knees, and ankles. They also occur on the scalp where they tend to be larger and less firm. They are also seen along the spine. Nodules range in size from tiny shotlike bodies to marble-sized protuberances. They are never transient and usually take weeks to disappear.

Nodules are most frequent in children with a prolonged active rheumatic carditis and in these patients they will often appear in recurrent crops. However the number of nodules cannot be correlated with the severity of the carditis (Baldwin et al., 1960). It is believed generally that patients with nodules have a poor prognosis, chiefly because this manifestation is virtually always associated with severe carditis. Massell and co-workers (1958) noted valvular damage in 91 per cent of patients with nodules. In the large series reported by Baldwin and her associates (1960), the mortality rate was higher in patients with nodules than that observed in children who had carditis without nodules.

Diagnosis

Nodules are of limited diagnostic value since overt evidence of carditis is almost always present in patients with this manifestation. If

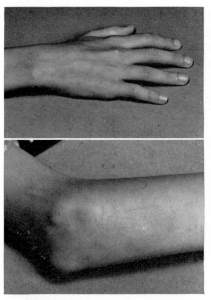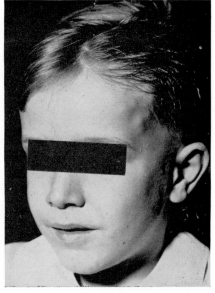

Figure 5. Subcutaneous nodules over bony prominences at different sites in 3 patients with active rheumatic fever.

there is no evidence of cardiac disease, the nodules are probably due to another condition, rheumatoid arthritis. In the latter disease, nodules are always associated with chronic joint involvement. Patients with rheumatic-like nodules without evidence of joint or heart disease have been reported, an occurrence which must be exceedingly rare (Taranta, 1962).

ERYTHEMA MARGINATUM

Erythema marginatum is the only significant cutaneous manifestation of rheumatic fever. It is considered a *major manifestation,* and occasionally its appearance can be most helpful in making a diagnosis in patients with suggestive signs of rheumatic fever such as abdominal pain, arthralgia, or questionable carditis. It is in many respects an unusual rheumatic manifestation. Like chorea, it often makes a delayed appearance. It usually cannot be correlated with other signs of rheumatic activity and it is unaffected by suppressive antirheumatic drugs. Although erythema marginatum has its highest incidence in acute rheumatic fever, it is not specific for this disease. It has been reported in drug reactions, in patients with glomerulonephritis, and in children in whom no etiologic factor could be found (Burke, 1955).

Incidence

Erythema marginatum is not an uncommon finding in rheumatic fever patients. It occurred in 65 of 497 children with initial or recurrent attacks of rheumatic fever in an international study (U.K. and U.S. Joint Report, 1955) and in 48 of 457 patients observed at The House of the Good Samaritan (Massell et al., 1958).

Clinical Findings

The lesions of erythema marginatum begin as small, pink or faintly red, slightly raised macules. The erythema extends outward causing a sharp margin, and the skin in the center returns to a normal color. The lesions frequently take the form of enlarging rings or wavy lines which coalesce (Fig. 6). When the lesions are predominantly circular, the term erythema annulare is used. They are not associated with itching and are often very transient. They occur most commonly over the trunk and inner aspects of the upper arm and thigh. Fair-skinned children are more likely to have erythema marginatum and the lesions can be accentuated by the application of heat.

Erythema marginatum often occurs in association with other rheumatic manifestations. Two groups of investigators have observed

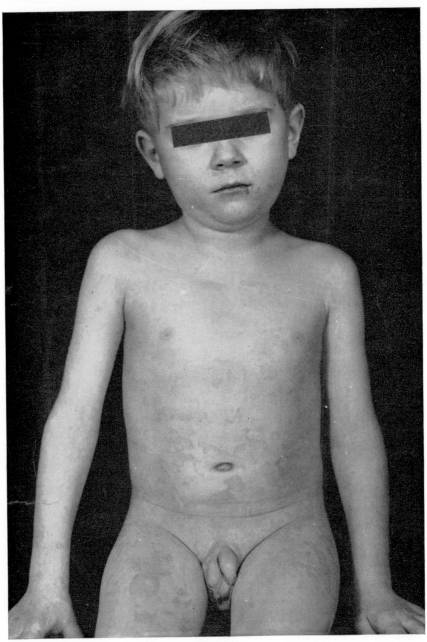

Figure 6. Erythema marginatum on the chest and abdomen of a boy 8 years of age.

erythema marginatum and subcutaneous nodules together in a somewhat larger number of patients than might be expected by chance (Massell et al., 1958; Feinstein and Spagnuolo, 1962). It has been the experience of most observers that carditis is commonly present in patients with erythema marginatum (Perry, 1937; Keil, 1938; Massell et al., 1958). However, rheumatic skin manifestations do not necessarily imply a poor prognosis, as has been suggested in the past (Wallgren, 1935).

Erythema marginatum may occur intermittently for many months in some patients, and, as has been noted, its course is uninfluenced by suppressive drugs. Since the skin lesions cannot usually be correlated with other signs or rheumatic activity, conservative management is not necessary if the other rheumatic manifestations have subsided.

Diagnosis

It is usually not difficult to identify erythema marginatum from the very characteristic appearance of the skin lesions. Circinate erythematous lesions may occur in drug reactions but they are usually papular and tend to be pruritic. The skin eruption seen in patients with rheumatoid arthritis is a pink macular rash without the characteristic sharp margins of erythema marginatum.

MINOR MANIFESTATIONS

Fever

Fever is almost always present at the onset of an acute attack of untreated rheumatic fever and it is considered a *minor manifestation*. The temperature ranges between 101 and 104° F., rarely higher. The fever has no characteristic pattern. Diurnal variations are common but large daily swings, such as are occasionally seen in children with rheumatoid arthritis, occur rarely in rheumatic fever. Children with a more insidious onset who usually have been ill for several weeks before they seek medical attention may have a low-grade fever, detectable only in the afternoon. Children with "pure" chorea are afebrile.

During the acute attack, fever usually decreases in a few days even without medication and then may become low-grade. Mildly elevated temperatures may persist for several weeks, but rarely longer. The sedimentation rate often remains elevated for variable periods of time after the temperature has returned to normal. If the temperature remains elevated it is usually an indication that activity of the rheumatic process has not subsided, and bed rest must be maintained and further medication considered.

In ambulatory children in whom the diagnosis is in doubt, it is sometimes necessary to have the mother take the temperature daily. This should be done only in very selected cases since normal diurnal variations tend to be overinterpreted. The mother should be instructed to have the child rest 15 minutes before the temperature is recorded. Rheumatic fever is rarely the cause of unexplained fever in children who have no other evidence of this disease.

Epistaxis

Formerly, in patients with severe carditis usually due to repeated attacks, nosebleeds were a common complication, not infrequently of such severity as to require transfusion. At the present time, when severe carditis is much less common, epistaxes are infrequent and mild. Feinstein and Spagnuolo (1962) reported an incidence of nosebleeds of 4 per cent in first attacks and of 9 per cent in recurrences.

Nosebleeds are common in children and in most instances are not associated with rheumatic fever. For this reason, extensive investigations to exclude rheumatic fever need not be carried out as a rule in children with nosebleeds.

Abdominal Pain

A complaint of abdominal pain not uncommonly is a symptom which brings the rheumatic child to the hospital or the physician. It may precede the initial attack or indicate the beginning of a recurrence in a known rheumatic. Physicians should be aware of the difficulty of differentiating the onset of rheumatic fever from acute appendicitis.

In young children the abdomen is often held rigid, and the site of the pain cannot be localized. Older children often complain of pain centered around the umbilicus. Not infrequently it is impossible to rule out the possibility of appendicitis. Rectal examination is sometimes helpful. If the child can be observed for a few hours, definite rheumatic symptoms may appear, such as a painful joint or erythema marginatum. At times an unusual tachycardia, poor heart sounds, or a suspicious murmur may be noted. The temperature is usually higher in rheumatic fever than in appendicitis. In the latter the onset of pain is often abrupt and vomiting is common. The white blood count is not helpful since it is elevated in appendicitis as well as in rheumatic fever. The most useful laboratory test is the sedimentation rate which is usually significantly elevated in rheumatic fever and normal or only slightly accelerated in appendicitis. If the findings remain equivocal, a surgical consultation may be necessary. If a serious doubt remains, it is better to remove a normal appendix than to risk rupture and generalized peritonitis.

Abdominal pain following the onset of acute polyarthritis is uncommon. It may occur in children with carditis and congestive heart failure, although pain in the hepatic region occurs less frequently in children with cardiac decompensation than in adults. Occasionally pleuritis or pericarditis may cause referred pain to the upper abdomen. Chronic abdominal symptoms during the course of rheumatic fever are exceedingly rare and are likely to be due to nonrheumatic causes including complications of treatment such as steroids.

"Rheumatic" Pneumonia

Pneumonia due specifically to the rheumatic inflammatory process ("rheumatic" pneumonia) may occur during the course of severe pancarditis. There is considerable disagreement, however, about the incidence of this complication. Indeed, some observers even doubt its existence (Feinstein and Spagnuolo, 1962). Brown and co-workers (1958) summarized many of the older published clinical reports and found that the incidence of pneumonia in rheumatic subjects varied between 1 and 27.8 per cent. In many instances, however, the etiology of the pneumonia could not be ascertained from the information available. In a more recent study, Goldring and associates (1958) collected 28 cases of "rheumatic" pneumonia over an 8 year period and found an overall incidence of 62 per cent among 87 children who died from rheumatic fever between 1919 and 1954.

Differences of opinion about the incidence and existence of "rheumatic" pneumonia occur because there are no characteristic pathologic, clinical, or roentgenographic findings on which to base the diagnosis. The lungs have a hemorrhagic appearance. Alveoli contain red blood cells, fibrin, and hemosiderin deposits and occasionally a hyaline membrane. None of these changes are specific for rheumatic fever. Rich and Gregory (1943) have likened the changes to those of an anaphylactic pneumonia presumably due to a vascular injury. The physical findings over the lung fields are sparse and when present cannot be distinguished from the signs associated with congestive failure. Since "rheumatic" pneumonia occurs chiefly in children with severe carditis, cardiac decompensation is frequently also present. Some observers have stressed the diagnostic value of the chest roentgenogram. Schwedel (1947) described a characteristic hilar distribution and Reinmann (1954) as well as Caffey (1950) mention the patchy, shifting nature of the infiltrates.

Our own experience suggests that "rheumatic" pneumonia is uncommon and that it cannot be diagnosed clinically. We have observed children with severe carditis in whom shifting areas of pulmonary infiltration were noted on the chest x-ray that did not respond to antimicrobial agents and that cleared only as the acute stage of rheumatic fever subsided. However, in none of these children could a viral pneumonitis be excluded.

Chapter Seven

LABORATORY FINDINGS

Laboratory findings which are helpful in the diagnosis and management of acute rheumatic fever fall into two groups: (1) studies confirmatory of a preceding streptococcal infection and (2) acute phase reactions for the evaluation of the inflammatory process during the active stage of the disease. None of these tests is specific for rheumatic fever. The lack of a specific diagnostic test is a real handicap when the clinical manifestations are not typical. Nevertheless, the laboratory procedures which are available are often an aid in the diagnosis and management of the disease (Wood and McCarty, 1954).

EVIDENCE OF A PRECEDING STREPTOCOCCAL INFECTION

The role of group A streptococci in the etiology of rheumatic fever is so firmly established that the diagnosis of rheumatic fever is often in doubt if no laboratory evidence of an antecedent streptococcal pharyngitis is demonstrable. However, even if proof of such an infection is obtained, it is not in itself sufficient to establish the diagnosis of rheumatic fever and must be correlated with clinical findings.

Bacteriologic Studies

At the time the child is first seen with rheumatic manifestations group A streptococci are demonstrable in throat cultures in only about 25 per cent of the patients. During the usual latent period of 1 to 3 weeks between the attack of pharyngitis and the appearance of rheumatic symptoms, the streptococci often disappear spontaneously or fail to grow because antimicrobial medication has been given. Furthermore, even if a positive culture is obtained, it is impossible to be sure that the streptococci isolated represent a recent infection, since children not infrequently are chronic carriers of these organisms. Bacteriologic studies therefore are of limited value.

Immunologic Studies

Reliable evidence of a preceding streptococcal infection can be obtained more readily by tests for streptococcal antibodies than by the isolation of streptococci from the pharynx. Of the various tests available for this purpose the antistreptolysin O (ASO) determination is the most useful. The antigen, streptolysin O, is commercially available and the procedure can be performed by most laboratories with reliable results. The highest dilution of the patient's serum that inhibits lysis of red blood cells by one unit of streptolysin O is the end point. The ASO titer is expressed in units as the reciprocal of the end-point dilution. The series of dilutions most commonly used results in the following progression of titers: 12, 50, 100, 125, 166, 250, 333, 500, 625, 833, 1250, and 2500 (Rantz and Randall, 1945).

The normal ASO titer varies with age, geographic area, and other factors (Rantz et al., 1948; Saslaw and Streitfield, 1959). The distribution of ASO titers in one metropolitan pediatric population is shown in Figure 7. The ASO titer increases from infancy and the highest levels are found in the school-age population. Titers as high as 250 units are common in well children aged 6 to 14 years who live in the north temperate zone.

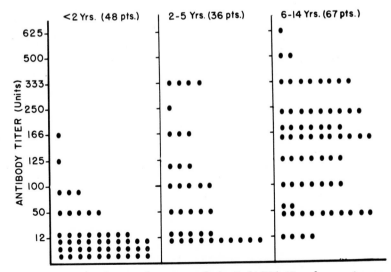

Figure 7. Distribution of antistreptolysin O (ASO) titers by age in asymptomatic children from a clinic population. (Adapted from Markowitz et al., 1965.)

In this age group a single titer of 333 units is considered borderline and a titer of 500 units is considered indicative of a recent streptococcal infection. A single low or borderline titer does not exclude a streptococcal infection. Regardless of the initial level, a rise or fall in titer of two or more increments (tube dilutions) in serial specimens is considered significant. In patients in whom the results are equivocal, it is best to perform the test on serial specimens simultaneously.

A rise in the ASO titer can be demonstrated in 75 to 85 per cent of patients following untreated streptococcal upper respiratory infections. The titer usually rises within 1 to 2 weeks and increases until a maximal level is reached 3 to 5 weeks after the infection. It remains elevated for a variable time and declines gradually to preinfection levels over a period of months. Penicillin therapy may modify the ASO response if given early in the course of the infection and in sufficient amount to eradicate the organisms (Kilbourne and Loge, 1948). Cortisone also may cause a delay in the development of antibody (Hahn et al., 1951).

Seventy-five to 85 per cent of patients with acute rheumatic fever have elevated ASO titers. The distribution of the maximal titers among patients with acute rheumatic fever, patients with uncomplicated streptococcal infections, and "well" children is shown in Figure 8. Approxi-

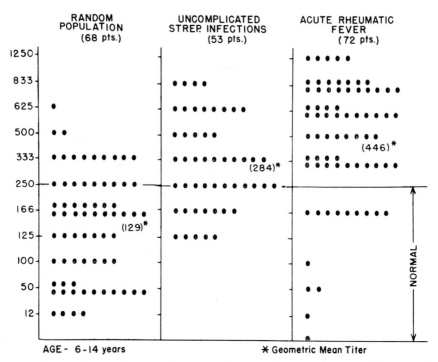

Figure 8. Distribution of antistreptolysin O (ASO) titers in children aged 6 to 14 in (1) a random population, (2) following uncomplicated streptococcal infections and (3) in acute rheumatic fever.

mately the same percentage of patients with uncomplicated streptococcal infections and with acute rheumatic fever have elevated titers. Titers tend to be higher in rheumatic patients than in children with uncomplicated streptococcal infections. There is, however, considerable overlap and the magnitude of the titer is not by itself diagnostic of rheumatic fever.

A single low or borderline ASO titer does not exclude acute rheumatic fever. In rheumatic subjects, there is occasionally a delay in the rise which may become apparent subsequently. When the results are equivocal, tests should be repeated at weekly intervals. Although the possible suppressive role of previous antibiotic therapy on the ASO titer must be considered, the titer in rheumatic patients is rarely affected, because if adequate doses of penicillin had been given, rheumatic fever would probably have been prevented.

It has been repeatedly observed both in epidemic as well as sporadic cases of streptococcal pharyngitis that in about 20 per cent of the patients no rise in the ASO titer occurs. This is true of uncomplicated streptococcal upper respiratory infections as well as in those followed by rheumatic fever. However, if in addition to the ASO the antibody responses to other enzymes produced by group A streptococci, such as hyaluronidase, streptokinase, DPNase, and DNase, are studied, evidence of a preceding streptococcal infection can be obtained in 95 per cent of patients with acute rheumatic fever (Stollerman, 1956) (Fig. 9). Satisfactory materials are available commercially to test for streptococcal hyaluronidase antibodies. Although the determinations of anti-DPNase and anti-DNase

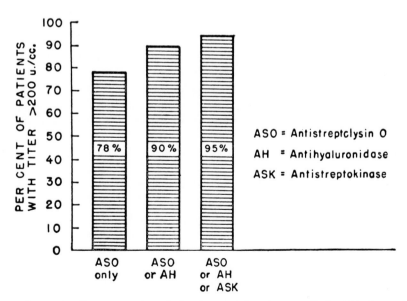

Figure 9.   Streptococcal antibody titers in 88 patients studied within 2 months of onset of rheumatic fever. (From Stollerman et al.: Amer. J. Med. 20:163, 1956.)

antibodies have been recommended as good secondary procedures, these tests are still difficult to perform in routine laboratories, and if important, should be done in special centers organized for streptococcal research. If a battery of streptococcal antibody determinations is carried out on serial specimens and fails to show significant elevations in titer, the diagnosis of acute rheumatic fever remains doubtful.

Streptococcal antibodies are rarely elevated in patients who are first observed several months after the onset of acute rheumatic fever and in those with chronic rheumatic heart disease. Since chorea is a late sequel of streptococcal infections, antibodies are often within the normal range in children with this manifestation. The rate of fall of antibody titers bears no relationship to the clinical course of the disease or to the prognosis. However, frequent determinations of streptococcal antibodies in rheumatic patients receiving continuous prophylaxis are useful as a means of detecting asymptomatic streptococcal infections and to rule out the possibility that subclinical attacks of rheumatic fever may have occurred.

ACUTE PHASE REACTANTS

General Considerations

A number of tests have been utilized to measure the presence and the degree of inflammation in patients with rheumatic fever: leukocyte count, erythrocyte sedimentation rate, C-reactive protein, serum mucoprotein, Weltmann reaction, serum hexosamine, and others. Leukocyte counts are too variable to be of value. The serum mucoprotein and other tests have not gained wide usage (Kelley et al., 1950). The two acute phase procedures most commonly used in rheumatic patients are the erythrocyte sedimentation rate (ESR) and the C-reactive protein (CRP).

It is well known that the acute phase reactants are abnormal in a wide variety of inflammatory conditions and that neither the ESR nor the CRP is specific for rheumatic fever. These tests are therefore of secondary importance as diagnostic tools. In certain cases, however, the CRP and ESR are helpful. In patients with vague complaints suggestive of rheumatic fever, a normal CRP or ESR makes it unlikely that symptoms are rheumatic. On the other hand, if in such cases these tests are unequivocally abnormal, these children should be examined at regular intervals because overt manifestations of rheumatic fever may develop. In the differential diagnosis of acute appendicitis from the abdominal pain occurring at the onset of a rheumatic attack, an elevated ESR or positive CRP make the diagnosis of rheumatic fever more likely. During streptococcal pharyngitis and also during other intercurrent upper respiratory infections the CRP and ESR are frequently abnormal. These infections are usually self-limited and the acute phase reactants return to normal promptly. Even in patients with streptococcal pharyngitis who subsequently develop rheumatic fever, the ESR and CRP are normal during the asymptomatic latent period, and only become positive at the time that the rheumatic manifestations appear. If following a proven streptococcal upper respiratory infection the ESR remains elevated for longer than a month, the patient should be followed to be sure that he is not experiencing an attack of subclinical rheumatic fever which after several weeks may become apparent by definite signs of heart disease. In patients with overt acute rheumatic fever once the acute manifestations are controlled, the CRP and ESR are useful in determining the persistence of rheumatic activity and in the medical management of the patient.

Erythrocyte Sedimentation Rate

The inflammatory process increases substances in the plasma which causes an augmentation in rouleau formation of red blood cells and speeds their fall in blood prevented from coagulating by various means. The speed of fall has been measured by a number of techniques. The Westergren and the Wintrobe methods are employed most commonly. The longer tube used with the Westergren technique provides a wider range between normal and abnormal values, and the results are not affected by anemia. The upper limit of normal is between 10 and 20 mm. in one hour. Until recently with the Wintrobe technique a correction for anemia was recommended but this is no longer necessary (Wintrobe, 1956). The upper limit of normal by the uncorrected Wintrobe method is 20 mm. per hour. The sedimentation rate may be modified by sicklemia and by changes which occur in the plasma proteins as a result of heart failure, liver disease, nephrosis, and other conditions.

The ESR is almost always abnormal in patients with untreated acute rheumatic fever. In children with "pure" chorea, on the other hand, it is usually normal. The magnitude of the increase in the ESR is proportionate to the intensity of the inflammatory reaction but bears no relationship to the site involved. The elevation of the ESR is often as striking in patients with joint involvement as in those with severe pancarditis. In children in whom the development of carditis has been insidious, the ESR not infrequently is only slightly increased. Indeed in patients with heart failure the ESR may be normal, presumably because fibrinogen production by the liver is decreased because of passive congestion.

It is not uncommon for the ESR to remain elevated for 6 weeks to 3 months following an untreated attack of acute rheumatic fever. Antiinflammatory agents such as salicylates and steroids lower the ESR. The speed with which it returns toward normal depends on the intensity of the inflammatory reaction and the dosage and type of anti-inflammatory drug. In general, steroids suppress the ESR somewhat more rapidly than salicylates. Although suppression of the acute phase reactants by anti-inflammatory agents usually coincides with a reduction in fever and the exudative manifestations in patients with significant carditis, the ESR usually does not correlate with changes in the cardiac findings. Thus the ESR may have returned to normal even though clinical evidence of active carditis persists. If the anti-inflammatory drugs are discontinued before the rheumatic process has run its course, the ESR rebounds and then usually returns gradually to normal. Rarely the ESR remains elevated for more than 6 months. The significance of this finding is not understood. Taranta and his associates (1962) have followed a number of patients with an elevated ESR for several years and their cardiac status remained unchanged.

Once the base line of the ESR is established in children with chronic rheumatic heart disease, determinations of the sedimentation rate need not be done routinely unless an exacerbation of symptoms occurs or a recurrence is suspected. It is not uncommon for an elevated ESR to persist in overweight children and in adolescents (Harris, 1945). Because of the reaction at the site of injection, the ESR may become elevated in patients receiving prophylactic injections of benzathine penicillin (Haas et al., 1957).

C-reactive Protein

C-reactive protein (CRP) is so called because it was first recognized as a substance which reacted with the C-polysaccharide of the pneumococcus (Tillet and Francis, 1930). The CRP is a unique protein not normally present in the blood. It appears promptly during the course of any inflammatory condition. The CRP protein is antigenic and highly specific antiserum is available commercially. This protein has been characterized as a beta globulin (Wood et al., 1954). The CRP is measured semiquantitatively by the amount of precipitate formed in a capillary tube when the patient's serum is added to the specific rabbit antiserum (Anderson and McCarty, 1950). Strong reactions may be visible within one hour, but weak reactions often require 24 hours. It is a useful additional acute phase test and has certain advantages over the ESR. One of the chief limitations of the ESR is that normal values are poorly defined; even a slightly positive CRP is significant.

The CRP, like the ESR, is nonspecific. During the acute stage both the CRP and the ESR are positive, but the CRP becomes normal more rapidly following the administration of anti-inflammatory medication than the ESR. The CRP usually remains positive in patients with active carditis who develop congestive heart failure, whereas the ESR may be normal. The CRP may also be abnormal in patients with congestive failure due to noninflammatory causes (Elster et al., 1956). In patients with rebounds following the withdrawal of suppressive drugs, the ESR is often elevated but the CRP remains normal. If the CRP is positive, it suggests that a flare-up of clinical manifestations is likely (Taranta et al., 1962). The CRP, like the ESR, is normal in patients with "pure" chorea.

In the opinion of several observers the CRP reflects rheumatic activity more precisely than the ESR, because it is determined by a specific immune reaction to a single protein (Anderson and McCarty, 1950; Ziegra and Kuttner, 1951; Stollerman et al., 1953). The ESR, on the other hand, depends on a number of different factors such as anemia and changes in serum proteins which vary from patient to patient. Neither the CRP nor ESR can detect underlying disease activity in patients in whom the clinical signs have been suppressed by anti-inflammatory medication. Elster and Wood (1955) observed no correlation with either the CRP or the ESR and the occurrence of Aschoff bodies in the left auricular appendage. A specific diagnostic test for rheumatic activity has so far not been devised.

MISCELLANEOUS LABORATORY FINDINGS

Anemia

Anemia of a mild to moderate degree occurs commonly in acute rheumatic fever. In patients with severe carditis, pallor is often striking. The anemia usually improves gradually as the inflammatory process subsides. Persistence of anemia is often a sign that rheumatic inflammation is still present.

Severe and repeated epistaxes may increase the anemia but are not the sole cause. Hubbard and McKee (1939) thought that the anemia was due to a depression of erythropoiesis by the inflammatory process. Reinhold (1954) suggested that hemolysis may play a role. Cochran (1951) and Mauer (1961) have shown that in the early stages of rheumatic fever there is an increase in plasma volume which decreases the red blood cell mass and is responsible for the low hematocrit levels. In the studies described by Mauer, however, some patients had decreased erythropoiesis and others a shortened survival time of the erythrocytes. It seems likely therefore that more than one factor may contribute to the development of anemia.

Serum Oxaloacetic Transaminase

Serum glutamic oxaloacetic transaminase (SGOT) is elevated in the presence of acute tissue damage and studies of this enzyme have been of value in patients with acute myocardial infarction. The SGOT has also been found to be elevated in patients with acute rheumatic fever (Nydick et al., 1955; Massie and Stahlman, 1958). However the enzyme levels are not consistently elevated in patients with acute rheumatic carditis and there is no correlation with the course of the disease. It is the impression of most observers that SGOT studies are of little or no value in rheumatic fever.

Serum Proteins

The serum gamma globulin is usually elevated in patients with acute rheumatic fever. The increase in gamma globulin is thought to be due chiefly to the rise in streptococcal antibodies and is not directly related to the rheumatic inflammation (Anderson et al., 1948). Electrophoretic studies have shown that in addition to the gamma globulin, a rise in alpha 1, alpha 2, and beta globulin may also occur (Kroop et al., 1954). Immunoelectrophoretic studies have shown that the major portion of the gamma globulin in rheumatic subjects is 7S. Hypergammaglobulinemia was also present in the families of the rheumatic patients (Bernstein and Allerhand, 1962).

An unusually high incidence of mesenchymal or collagen disease has been reported in patients with agammaglobulinemia. The associated conditions include rheumatoid arthritis, scleroderma, and dermatomyositis (Good and Gabrielson, 1964). It is of interest, however, that there is no record of rheumatic fever occurring in any of the patients with gamma globulin deficiencies despite their marked susceptibility to streptococcal infections.

Urinary 5-Methoxytryptamine

Haddox and Saslaw (1963) have reported the occurrence of an abnormal product of tryptophan metabolism, 5-methoxytryptamine, in the urine of rheumatic subjects and have suggested that this finding may be a useful aid in diagnosis. Their observations require confirmation.

Chapter Eight

RADIOGRAPHIC AND ELECTROCARDIOGRAPHIC FINDINGS

The roentgenogram and the electrocardiogram are often useful in the diagnosis of acute rheumatic fever. In this chapter only the significant findings observed during the *acute* attack will be discussed. Changes in the roentgenograms and electrocardiograms of patients with established valvular lesions are discussed in the chapter on chronic rheumatic heart disease (page 149).

RADIOGRAPHY

Arthritis

Occasionally, at the onset of rheumatic fever, the signs and symptoms are limited to one joint. In such patients, radiographic examination of the joint and surrounding tissues is often desirable to exclude trauma, septic arthritis, osteomyelitis, or other conditions. On the other hand, in children with polyarthritis, x-rays of the joints do not usually aid in the diagnosis and are not necessary. If the joint symptoms are severe, it may not be possible to obtain adequate x-rays of the heart because the patient is unable to stand. Radiologic examination of the heart should be deferred until the joint symptoms have been controlled or have diminished.

Carditis

Roentgenograms are particularly useful to detect slight to moderate degrees of cardiac enlargement. The detection of cardiomegaly is of

71

considerable importance since it may confirm the diagnosis of carditis in doubtful cases. Posteroanterior and oblique views of the chest should be obtained. Measurements should be made of the transverse diameter of the heart and the greatest horizontal distance between the inner border of the ribs at the level of the diaphragm domes. The diameter of the heart as compared to the internal chest diameter is the cardiothoracic ratio. This ratio is normally less than 0.5. Care must be taken against overinterpretation of x-ray findings. The heart size varies with body build and the range of normal is considerable. When the enlargement is equivocal, serial examinations may be necessary before a final decision can be reached. A significant decrease in the size of the heart shadow as the patient improves will afford retrospective evidence of enlargement (Fig. 10).

Cardiac enlargement may be due to dilatation, pre-existing heart disease, or pericardial effusion. Acute rheumatic myocarditis does not cause a characteristic cardiac contour. The cardiothoracic ratio is increased and there is fullness of the left cardiac border (Fig. 11). In severe myocarditis the heart assumes a globular shape and is enlarged both to the left and right of the sternum. The differentiation between pericardial effusion and generalized enlargement due to dilatation may be particularly difficult. Small amounts of effusion can rarely be detected even on x-ray. An increase in the acuteness of the cardiodiaphragmatic angles is a suggestive sign. A rapid increase in size usually signifies effusion. If the effusion is large, the cardiac silhouette has a water-bottle ("gourd-shaped") configuration when the patient is in the erect position (Fig. 12). A large cardiac shadow with clear lung fields and normal vascular markings should suggest an effusion, in contrast to the dilated heart with prominent vascular markings characteristic of congestive heart failure. A cardiac scan may be helpful in distinguishing effusion from dilatation (Fig. 12). Serial x-ray examinations are also often helpful. A rapid diminution in the size of the cardiac shadow is more likely to occur when effusion is present (Fig. 13). After the effusion disappears, enlargement of the heart due to residual myocarditis or pre-existing valvular disease may become apparent.

The degree of enlargement is a valuable index of severity and is a useful parameter in observing the course of the patient. In patients with acute rheumatic fever, cardiac enlargement is due chiefly to myocarditis rather than valvular damage. However, active carditis may be present even though the heart size is normal. In the majority of patients with enlargement, the heart size usually returns to normal gradually over a period of weeks or months. It is not uncommon to note improvement in size even though signs of valvular damage persist (see Fig. 11). Progressive enlargement is an unequivocal sign of active rheumatic carditis (Fig. 14). If the heart remains enlarged, permanent cardiac damage is likely. However, there are occasions when the heart continues to be

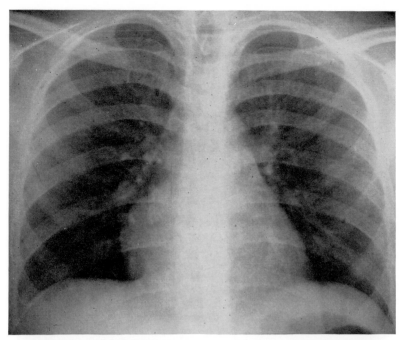

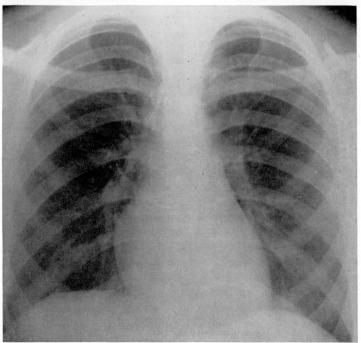

Figure 10. Posteroanterior views of an 11 year old girl with acute rheumatic fever with questionable clinical signs of carditis. Her first film (top) suggested mild cardiac enlargement. A marked decrease in heart size was noted in the film taken 3 weeks later (bottom), indicating that dilatation of the heart was unequivocally present initially.

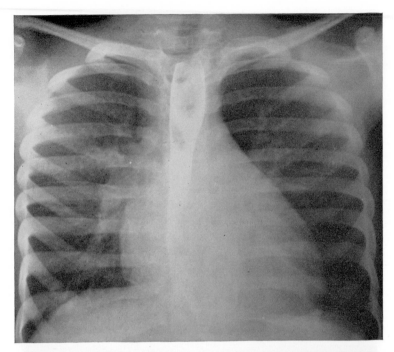

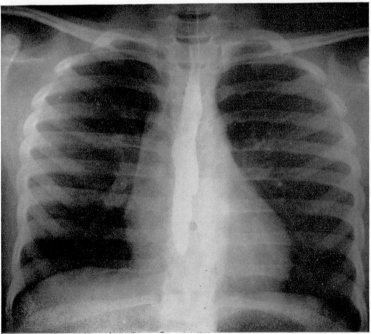

Figure 11. Posteroanterior views of a 10 year old girl with a first attack of acute rheumatic fever with myocarditis and mitral regurgitation. The top view was taken at the onset of the attack and shows generalized cardiac enlargement. The bottom view was taken 4 months later. The heart has returned to normal in size, although the murmur of mitral regurgitation is still present.

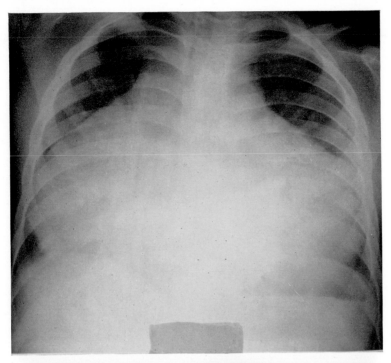

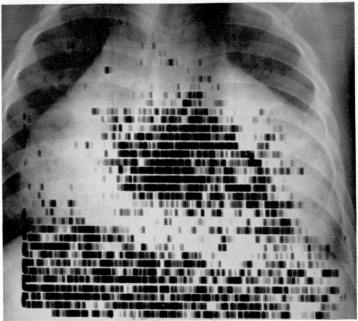

Figure 12. Posteroanterior views of the chest of an 11 year old Negro boy with rheumatic heart disease, a pericardial friction rub, aortic and mitral insufficiency, and sickle cell anemia. The top film demonstrates the huge "water-bottle" cardiac shadow. The bottom film was taken 2 days later, following injection of I^{131} cholografin, and shows the discrepancy between the scanning image of the cardiac blood pool and the cardiac silhouette caused by the accumulation of pericardial fluid.

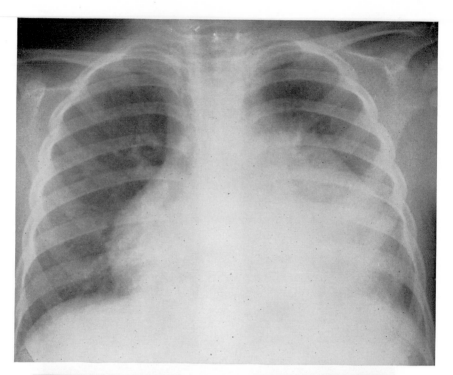

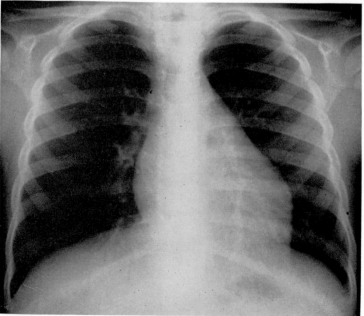

Figure 13. Posteroanterior views of a 5 year old boy with acute rheumatic fever and pericarditis. The top film shows the cardiac silhouette on admission. The bottom film was taken after 1 week of suppressive therapy. The rapid change in size is characteristic of pericardial effusion.

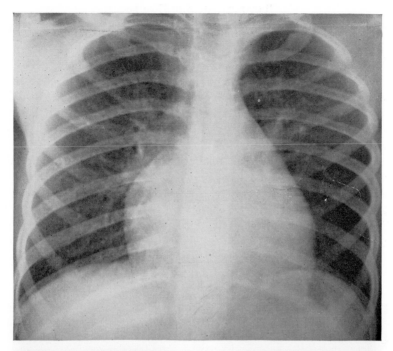

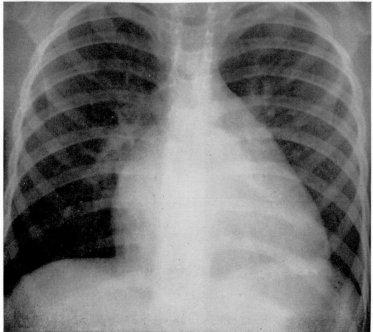

Figure 14. Posteroanterior views of a 6 year old girl with acute rheumatic fever and myocarditis. The top view was taken at the onset of the attack and shows slight cardiac enlargement. The bottom view was taken 3 months later. Further cardiac enlargement had occurred and there was clinical and laboratory evidence of persistent rheumatic activity.

slightly enlarged even though all other signs have become stabilized. In such children, subsequent growth of the chest will often return the cardiothoracic ratio to normal limits (Taussig and Goldenberg, 1941).

Wilson (1960) has advocated fluoroscopic examination to determine the angle at which the left ventricle clears the spine as a means of detecting early enlargement of this chamber in patients with acute rheumatic fever. Using a turntable, she found that 97 per cent of normal children have an angle of clearance of less than 55 degrees but in the majority of patients with left ventricular enlargement the angle of clearance is increased. This technique is useful in children with high diaphragms and transverse hearts, in whom cardiac enlargement is suspected (Kuttner and Reyersbach, 1939). However, most investigators have not found this method reliable enough for general use because of the wide range of normal variation and the technical difficulties in obtaining an accurate measurement of the angle of clearance (Ravin and Nice, 1952). Enlargement of the left ventricle can usually be detected equally well in the

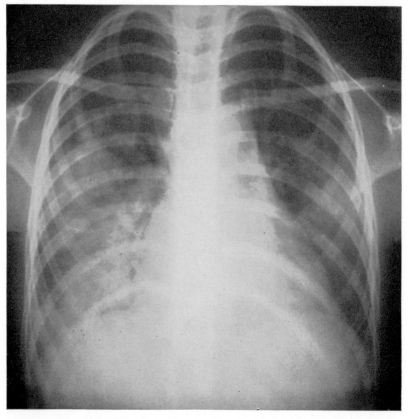

Figure 15.   Chest film of an 11 year old girl with fulminant rheumatic carditis leading rapidly to death. The heart is enlarged. There are many confluent irregular densities in the lung fields due to pulmonary edema.

left anterior oblique view. This provides a permanent record and exposes the patient to less radiation than fluoroscopic examination.

Pulmonary Findings

When congestive heart failure is present, the hilar shadows are prominent and coarse linear streaks radiate into the bases. Confluent irregular densities in the middle and lower lung fields indicate pulmonary edema (Fig. 15).

"Rheumatic" pneumonitis occurs in a small percentage of severely ill children. It is difficult to distinguish this entity from pulmonary edema. Patchy areas of infiltration throughout the lung fields suggest pneumonitis. Caffey (1950) has emphasized the fleeting migratory nature of the radiographic findings. A pleural reaction and effusion may also occur.

ELECTROCARDIOGRAPHY

Electrocardiographic abnormalities in acute rheumatic fever are of three general varieties: (1) disturbances in conduction, (2) changes associated with myocarditis, and (3) abnormalities secondary to pericardial involvement. There is no characteristic pattern for acute rheumatic fever and the diagnosis should never be made on the basis of electrocardiographic findings alone. Furthermore, there is no correlation between the severity of the attack and the electrocardiographic changes, and neither the course of the acute attack nor the development of valvular or myocardial damage can be predicted from the electrocardiogram.

Conduction Disturbances

The most common finding noted in acute rheumatic fever is a delay in atrioventricular (AV) conduction, as evidenced usually by a prolonged PR interval. The PR interval is defined as the longest interval in any of the 6 bipolar or unipolar extremity leads from the beginning of the P wave to the beginning of the QRS complex, whether represented by a Q wave or an R wave. The PR interval varies with age and heart rate and normal values have been tabulated in standard tables (Ashman and Hull, 1941; Alimurung and Massell, 1956). Care must be taken not to overinterpret minor differences in the PR interval as compared to normal standards. In a single tracing a PR interval of more than 0.20 second is indicative of first degree heart block (Fig. 16A). If the PR interval is less than 0.20 second, the diagnosis of heart block can be made only if a significant change occurs in serial electrocardiograms. In general, an increase or decrease of 0.04 second in the PR interval in tracings with

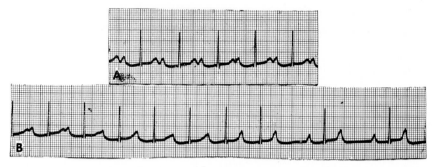

Figure 16. Heart block in acute rheumatic fever. A, First degree AV block with a PR interval of 0.36 second. B, Wenckebach phenomenon: slowly progressing PR intervals from 0.36 second to 0.44 second followed by a dropped beat. After the dropped beat, first and second degree heart block appears.

comparable rates is considered significant. Transient changes in the PR interval occur frequently. Recently, Mirowski and co-workers (1964) suggested that AV conduction should be expressed in terms of a ratio (the PR index) between the actual PR interval (numerator) and the upper limit of normal for the given age and the heart rate (denominator) (Fig. 17). The PR index gives an accurate method for the comparison of the AV conduction in electrocardiograms obtained from children of different ages with different heart rates.

First degree heart block occurs in 25 to 40 per cent of patients during the acute stage of rheumatic fever. The incidence of first degree heart block among acute rheumatic fever subjects, normal children, and patients with nonrheumatic illnesses studied at the Johns Hopkins Hospital is shown in Table 9. This table shows that occasionally the PR interval is prolonged in a variety of disorders and even in a small percentage of apparently normal children. Prolongation of the PR interval has been

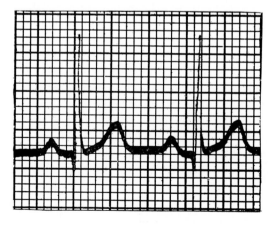

Figure 17. Determination of the PR index. In this example, the PR interval measures 0.15 second and the heart rate is 93 per minute. The upper limit of normal for this age (8 years) and heart rate, according to Ashman and Hull's tables, is 0.16. The PR index is, therefore, 0.15/0.16 = 0.94. (From Mirowski et al.: Pediatrics 33:334, 1964.)

Table 9. Incidence of Heart Block in Normal Children, Nonrheumatic Illnesses, and Rheumatic Fever and Its Relationship to Rheumatic Heart Disease*

Group	No. of Cases	% Prolonged PR Interval	% Residual Heart Disease
Normal	50	2	—
Nonrheumatic Illnesses	64	4	—
Polyarthritis	46	33	0
Carditis	50	40	43

* Modified from data compiled by Mirowski et al. (1964).

reported in patients following a streptococcal sore throat and scarlet fever in the absence of rheumatic sequelae (Rantz et al., 1946; Levander-Lindgren, 1952). Therefore an AV conduction disturbance should not be considered a specific rheumatic manifestation. Nevertheless, because of the frequency with which a prolonged PR interval is found in rheumatic fever, occasionally it is helpful in establishing the diagnosis. For example, it is often difficult to be certain of the diagnosis in children with arthralgia, or with transient or mono-articular arthritis. The occurrence of first degree heart block de novo in these patients is an exceedingly useful finding and makes the diagnosis of rheumatic fever much more likely.

Other disturbances in AV conduction, such as progressive lengthening of the PR interval in the same tracing (Wenckebach phenomenon), complete heart block, and AV dissociation, may be observed (Fig. 16B). Nodal rhythm and premature contractions may occur. Auricular fibrillation occurs chiefly in patients with established organic heart disease.

The exact mechanism of delayed AV conduction in acute rheumatic fever is not known. It may be due to a heightened vagal tone since atropine has been observed to shorten the PR interval (Keith, 1938; Robinson, 1945). Contrary to a widely held belief, it is probably not related to myocardial inflammation. The incidence of AV conduction disturbances is not significantly greater in children with clinical evidence of cardiac involvement than in patients with polyarthritis alone (Feinstein and DiMassa, 1959; Mirowski et al., 1964). Prolonged AV conduction cannot be correlated with other signs of rheumatic activity. First degree heart block may persist for a long time in a small percentage of patients and has no prognostic significance (Reyersbach and Kuttner, 1940). It has been observed repeatedly that patients with abnormal electrocardiographic findings without clinical signs of carditis almost always recover completely and on follow-up examination usually have normal cardiac findings (Feinstein et al., 1964). These data suggest that an abnormality of AV conduction is not part of a generalized cardiac process and, of itself, bears no relationship to the ultimate prognosis of the patients.

Myocarditis

The presence of myocarditis is suggested by notched, flattened or inverted T waves in one or several leads in patients with acute rheumatic fever. In general, T wave changes occur much less frequently than AV conduction disturbances. They are frequently transient and are not particularly common even in children with overt carditis. Although these abnormalities may be due to myocardial or subepicardial involvement, they are not specific for rheumatic fever and are observed in other acute febrile conditions (Levander-Lindgren, 1952). In individuals with ill-defined

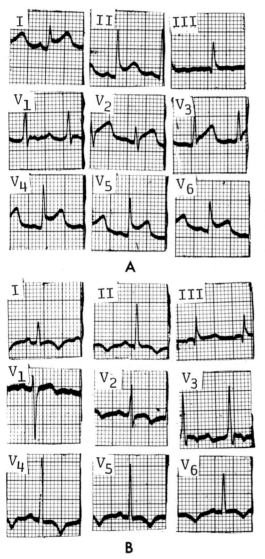

Figure 18. EKG tracings from a 10 year old girl with pericarditis. A, EKG at onset: marked elevation of ST segment in leads I, II, V₃, V₄, V₅, and V₆. B, EKG 2 weeks after onset: ST segments have returned to the iso-electric line, but T waves are inverted in leads I, II, and in all precordial leads from V₃ to V₆. (Courtesy of Dr. Harold H. Bix.)

illnesses a diagnosis of rheumatic myocarditis should not be made on the basis of T wave changes alone.

In the past several years investigators have suggested that the QT interval (electrical systole) is significantly prolonged in patients with myocarditis and that this finding is a sensitive indicator of active carditis (Taran and Szilagyi, 1952; Carmichael, 1955). A number of methods have been used to correct the QT interval for heart rate and other factors. As a result different surveys report divergent findings which make interpretation difficult. At the present time it is the consensus of most workers that although the QT interval may be prolonged in acute myocarditis, it is not a uniformly reliable indicator of acute carditis and cannot be correlated directly with inflammatory changes in the myocardium.

Pericarditis

Confirmatory evidence of pericarditis is frequently obtained in electrocardiographic tracings. The characteristic patterns associated with pericarditis are due to injury to the subepicardial portion of the myocardium. An upward deviation of the ST segments of more than 1 mm. in the three standard bipolar leads and of more than 2 mm. in the precordial leads is commonly seen. The ST segment changes occur early in the course of pericarditis (Fig. 18A). During the early stages the T waves may be normal but subsequently they often become flattened or inverted (Fig. 18B). Care must be taken against overinterpretation of minor ST segment elevations. They are common in children, especially in the transitional precordial leads. A large pericardial effusion is unusual in rheumatic fever but when it does occur, low voltage of the QRS complexes and the T waves may occur. Obvious clinical signs of pericarditis may be present without electrocardiographic changes.

Chapter Nine

DIFFERENTIAL DIAGNOSIS

Acute rheumatic fever is an illness characterized by a number of clinical features usually appearing in various combinations. The frequent occurrence of such combinations led Dr. T. Duckett Jones, in 1944, to formulate criteria for guidance in the diagnosis of acute rheumatic fever. There was not then, nor is there now, a single clinical sign or laboratory test which is pathognomonic for rheumatic fever. In the 20 years since the criteria were published, there have been no major advances in diagnostic procedures other than improved techniques for the determination of anti-streptococcal antibodies. The Jones criteria were modified in 1955 and are presently being revised, chiefly to emphasize the importance of establishing antecedent streptococcal infection in the diagnosis of rheumatic fever. According to the revised recommendations, two major criteria, or one major and two minor criteria, indicate a high probability of rheumatic fever, if supported by evidence of a preceding streptococcal infection. The criteria are listed in Table 10. The clinical and laboratory manifestations on which these criteria are based have been discussed in Chapters 6 through 8.

The Jones criteria have been generally accepted and are now widely used by physicians in this country and in Europe. They have proved to be extremely useful and when strictly applied, few patients are misdiagnosed. However, errors in diagnosis are still made. Two recent surveys have shown that slightly more than 10 per cent of patients referred to institutions for rheumatic children were incorrectly diagnosed (Feinstein et al., 1960; Grossman and Athreya, 1962). Incorrect diagnoses are also commonly encountered in consultation clinics. In a recent study, 35 per cent of patients referred with a history of rheumatic fever or rheumatic heart disease, or both, were improperly diagnosed (Blackman, 1963).

There are many reasons why rheumatic fever and rheumatic heart

Table 10. The Jones Criteria (Modified)[*]

Major Criteria	Minor Criteria
Carditis	Fever
Polyarthritis	Arthralgia
Chorea	Prolonged PR interval
Subcutaneous nodules	Increased ESR or CRP
Erythema marginatum	Preceding group A streptococcal infection
	Previous rheumatic fever or inactive rheumatic heart disease

[*] Mod. Conc. Cardiov. Dis. 24:291, 1955.

disease are misdiagnosed (Hallidie-Smith and Bywaters, 1958; Markowitz, 1960).

1. There are clinical syndromes which fulfill the criteria but are not due to rheumatic fever. Common examples are patients with polyarthritis due to miscellaneous causes, chiefly rheumatoid arthritis, in whom further observation usually provides the correct diagnosis.

2. Patients seen early in the course of a rheumatic attack may not meet the criteria initially and are incorrectly diagnosed until other rheumatic manifestations appear. For example, children with rheumatic abdominal pain are often thought to have appendicitis until arthritis or carditis develops.

3. Subacute rheumatic fever may be overlooked entirely if conclusions are based only on early and incomplete evidence. A mild attack of rheumatic fever may never meet the criteria.

4. Not infrequently children are seen late in the course of a genuine attack and would have fulfilled the criteria if the history and physical findings could have been substantiated. Such cases should be classified as probable rheumatic fever.

5. Patients may be incorrectly diagnosed because the history and physical findings are misinterpreted or for lack of a thorough investigation including evidence of an antecedent streptococcal infection.

6. The diagnosis of rheumatic heart disease may have been made on inadequate evidence.

Some of the difficulties in diagnosis are insurmountable and are due to limitations in the Jones criteria and the tremendous variability of the disease. The major source of errors is a misinterpretation of certain physical and laboratory findings which happen to fulfill the Jones criteria. In the following section the more common conditions which should be considered in the differential diagnosis of rheumatic fever and rheumatic heart disease are discussed with special emphasis on the common sources of errors.

Joint Diseases Simulating Rheumatic Fever

Polyarthritis. The distinctive feature of joint involvement in rheumatic fever is its migratory, transient nature. However, this feature may be mimicked by other diseases, especially rheumatoid arthritis. The joint symptoms of rheumatoid arthritis may initially respond to salicylates in a way similar to that observed in rheumatic fever. If pericarditis is present, it may confuse the picture further since pericardial inflammation may occur early in the course of both diseases. Laboratory aids are of little value, since tests for rheumatoid factor are usually negative in children and the acute phase reactants (ESR and CRP) are abnormal in both diseases. An elevated ASO titer favors a diagnosis of rheumatic fever. Usually the patient's course will clarify the problem. Recurrences of joint symptoms while the patient is receiving adequate salicylate therapy is often the first signal that the symptoms are due to rheumatoid arthritis. A high, intermittent fever occurs not uncommonly in rheumatoid disease and rarely in rheumatic fever. The chronic nature of the arthritis and the subsequent appearance of a salmon-pink, macular rash, splenomegaly, and lymphadenopathy definitely establishes the diagnosis of rheumatoid arthritis.

Polyarthritis may occur early in the course of periarteritis nodosa, lupus erythematosis, and dermatomyositis. The arthritic symptoms are usually mild and other characteristic features are either present or emerge as the patient is observed. Joint involvement may be a prominent feature of Henoch-Schönlein purpura and may sometimes precede the appearance of skin lesions. Since this condition not uncommonly follows an upper respiratory infection and may be accompanied by severe abdominal pain, differentiation from rheumatic fever is often difficult. The appearance of petechiae over the lower half of the body is typical of the Henoch-Schönlein syndrome. In the differential diagnosis of polyarthritis the exclusion of hypersensitivity reactions is important. The joint symptoms may be due to penicillin given for an antecedent respiratory infection or serum sickness (tetanus antitoxin). Angioneurotic edema and urticaria strongly favor the diagnosis of an allergic reaction.

Mono-articular Arthritis. Rheumatic fever beginning with involvement of a single joint poses a different set of diagnostic problems. A careful history, the presence of fever, positive acute phase reactants, and roentgenographic studies will help to exclude trauma. Mono-articular involvement is common in juvenile rheumatoid arthritis, but although there may be considerable swelling, tenderness usually is less marked than in rheumatic fever, and the systemic reaction minimal or absent. A more urgent and difficult problem in the acutely ill, toxic child is to distinguish between rheumatic fever and a septic process, within the joint or adjacent bony structures. Sepsis may cause identical local and systemic findings. If the diagnosis is in doubt, the joint should be aspirated without delay. Synovial fluid containing 100,000 or more cells per cubic mm. is diagnostic of a septic process. On the other hand, once a septic process has been excluded, it is advisable to withhold salicylates in order not to suppress the appearance of involvement of another joint which would establish the diagnosis of rheumatic fever.

Pain in the hip can be a particularly puzzling symptom in children and several conditions should be considered in the differential diagnosis (Monty, 1962). Acute transient synovitis of the hip joint is a common cause of pain and since it is often associated with fever and a history of a respiratory infection, it may be confused with rheumatic fever. Rheumatic fever is relatively uncommon in children aged 3 to 5 years, in contrast to transient synovitis which occurs not infrequently in this age period. The hip joint is usually less frequently involved than other large joints in patients with rheumatic fever. Synovitis of the hip is usually a self-limited condition of fairly short duration and the course of the illness does not resemble rheumatic fever. Chronic and recurrent hip pain may be due to Legg-Perthes disease or a slipped epiphysis and these diagnoses can be established by radiologic examination.

Cardiac Conditions Simulating Rheumatic Fever and Rheumatic Heart Disease

Innocent Murmurs. The frequent occurrence of innocent systolic heart murmurs in children has been repeatedly emphasized (Friedman et al., 1949; Gardiner and Keith, 1951; Fogel, 1957; Lessof and Brigden, 1957). Nevertheless, misinterpretation of this finding remains a major source of overdiagnosis. An apical systolic murmur discovered during a routine physical examination may lead to an erroneous diagnosis of rheumatic mitral regurgitation. If the murmur is loud and well referred to the axilla, or even to the back, it is often assumed that it must have pathologic significance. Innocent murmurs are not infrequently loud and widely transmitted in children. Another common misconception is that innocent murmurs diminish with exercise, when indeed the opposite is often true. During an intercurrent febrile illness a systolic murmur not previously noted may suggest acute rheumatic carditis. The "newness" or the changed quality of the murmur is caused by the fever and accompanying tachycardia. Furthermore, an ill child is usually examined in the supine position which tends to make an innocent murmur more readily audible.

The characteristics of innocent systolic murmurs have been described in detail (Wells, 1954; Fogel, 1957; Paulin and Maunheimer, 1957). Two types comprise 95 per cent of innocent murmurs in children: the parasternal and the pulmonic (Fogel, 1960). The parasternal murmur is Still's "physiologic bruit" (1918) heard best in the third or fourth intercostal space to the left of the sternal border. The intensity is usually maximal between the sternum and the apex and although sometimes audible at the apex and in the axilla, the murmur is loudest to the right of the midclavicular line inside the apex. The parasternal innocent murmur varies between grades I and III in intensity and occupies the early part of mid-

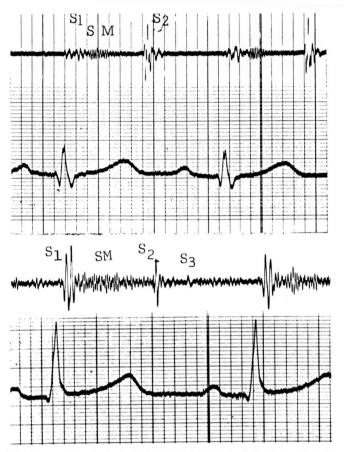

Figure 19. Oscillographic phonocardiograms recorded at the apex. *Top*: A 6 year old boy with a musical systolic murmur. The wave pattern is regular and occupies early midsystole. *Bottom*: An 8 year old girl with a pansystolic murmur of mitral regurgitation.

systole. It is the quality and not its loudness which differentiates the parasternal innocent from the organic murmur. The innocent murmur has a vibratory quality variously described as musical, groaning, or twanging-string. It is loudest in the recumbent position and is accentuated after exercise, excitement, or fever. Phonocardiographic tracings reveal a pattern which can be readily distinguished from the murmur of mitral regurgitation (Fig. 19). The mechanism of the musical innocent murmur is not fully understood. McKusick (1958) has suggested that it is due to triangulation of the pulmonary valve.

The pulmonic type of innocent systolic murmur occurs more frequently than the parasternal. It is an ejection murmur probably caused by the flow of blood from the right ventricle into the pulmonary artery. Because of its location the pulmonic type causes more confusion with

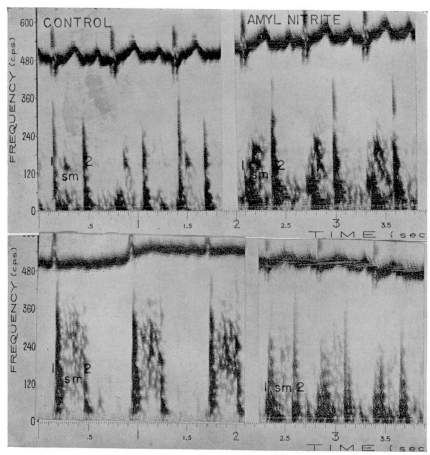

Figure 20. Comparative effect of amyl nitrite on innocent and mitral regurgitant murmurs recorded at the apex by spectral phonocardiography. *Top:* Innocent systolic murmur increases after inhalation of amyl nitrite. *Bottom:* Regurgitant systolic murmur decreases after inhalation of amyl nitrite. (Recordings courtesy of Dr. J. O'Neal Humphries.)

congenital than with rheumatic heart disease. This murmur is short and is heard best in the first part of systole. It is blowing and of moderate intensity, and it is usually heard maximally at the second left intercostal space. Occasionally it may even be heard at the apex. It varies in intensity, is accentuated by exercise, and is loudest when the child is recumbent.

The differentiation between innocent and organic murmurs can usually be made clinically by the experienced physician (Humphries and McKusick, 1962). However, there are occasions when an electrocardiogram and roentgenograms are indicated to reassure not only the parents but the physician as well. A phonocardiographic study may be helpful (Fig. 19). Pharmacologic agents also may aid in the differentiation (Paulin and Mannheimer, 1957). Vasoactive drugs such as amyl nitrite increase the intensity of innocent murmurs and decrease the intensity of organic mitral regurgitant murmurs (Fig. 20).

Myocarditis. Children with ill defined illnesses are sometimes mistakenly suspected of having rheumatic myocarditis on the basis of questionable evidence, especially if an innocent systolic murmur is present. Tachycardia is a common complaint by the referring physician or the parent. Careful evaluation will usually reveal that the increased pulse rate is due to apprehension or some other cause. Misinterpretation of normal variations of cardiac size and contour in the roentgenogram may also lead to an erroneous diagnosis of myocarditis. Similarly, minor changes in the electrocardiogram, particularly in the PR interval, ST segments, and T waves, are frequently assigned undue significance.

The differentiation between rheumatic fever and nonrheumatic myocarditis is seldom difficult because the latter is rarely associated with a significant murmur. Occasionally children between 3 and 6 years of age will present with a large heart, a gallop rhythm, a soft nondescript systolic murmur, and signs of congestive heart failure, and these signs suggest the possibility of a viral myocarditis. However, as cardiac function improves, often a regurgitant murmur characteristic of rheumatic heart disease becomes audible.

Pericarditis. A pericardial rub or effusion associated with evidence of myocarditis or valvulitis, or with other typical rheumatic manifestations, presents no diagnostic difficulty. Isolated pericarditis is rarely due to rheumatic fever and rheumatoid pericarditis or primary viral pericarditis (acute benign pericarditis) is more likely. Since rheumatoid pericarditis usually follows chronic joint disease, the diagnosis in most cases is not difficult. Occasionally pericarditis precedes arthritis and other rheumatoid manifestations (Lietman and Bywaters, 1963).

The differential diagnosis usually rests between rheumatic fever pericarditis and primary viral pericarditis (Friedman et al., 1952). A history of a preceding respiratory infection and vague pains in the extremities may be obtained in both conditions. The friction rub and effusion sometimes obscure heart murmurs and cardiac enlargement so that the diagnosis of rheumatic fever may not be possible until the pericarditis begins to subside. The clinical appearance of patients with primary viral pericarditis usually differs strikingly from that of children with rheumatic fever pericarditis. Patients with primary viral pericarditis are only mildly ill in contrast to children with rheumatic pericarditis. An elevated ASO titer favors the latter diagnosis. At times it is not possible to distinguish between these two conditions and, rarely, a combination of viral pericarditis and rheumatic heart disease may coexist (Woodward et al., 1960). If the diagnosis remains in doubt, antistreptococcal prophylaxis should be instituted and follow-up examinations performed until a definite diagnosis is established. Occasionally viral pericarditis in adults is associated with myocarditis and these patients may subsequently develop evidence of myocardial damage. The prognosis in children with primary viral pericarditis, on the other hand, is usually good.

Congenital Heart Disease. *Acute* rheumatic carditis is rarely mistaken for congenital heart disease. However, when a cardiac murmur due to a congenital lesion is first discovered during the course of an intercurrent febrile illness in a child of school age, rheumatic carditis may be suspected. This is especially true if, in addition to the murmur, the heart sounds are overactive and early signs of congestive failure are present. Careful evaluation of the murmur and the roentgenographic and electrocardiographic findings obtained on recovery from the infection will usually clarify the diagnosis.

Chronic rheumatic valvular disease, however, is more commonly confused with congenital heart disease. The systolic murmur of a ventricular septal defect with a small left to right shunt may resemble the murmur of mild mitral regurgitation. Usually the murmur of a ventricular septal defect is more clearly heard along the left sternal border and is more likely to be associated with a thrill. In children with large left to right shunts the differentiation from mitral regurgitation presents less of a problem.

Patent ductus arteriosus, coarctation of the aorta, and other congenital defects causing left ventricular enlargement may be associated with mitral regurgitation. This is due to dilatation of the mitral ring and to a change in orientation of the chordae and papillary muscles which prevents them from holding the cusps in proper position (Levy and Edwards, 1962).

It is more difficult to distinguish mitral incompetence of rheumatic valvular disease from congenital defects of the mitral valve. Many such defects have been described (Table 11). When the mitral defect is part of a complex of cardiac anomalies, as for example in ostium primum defects, the diagnosis can usually be made from the history, the associated clinical features, and the x-ray and electrocardiographic findings (Keith, 1962). However, it is difficult to exclude rheumatic heart disease when there is an isolated defect of the mitral valve. This diagnostic dilemma arises in children over 2 years of age who have the classic findings of mitral regurgitation without a history of rheumatic fever. They

Table 11.   Congenital Cardiac Lesions Associated with
Mitral Regurgitation

Endocardial cushion defects
Corrected transposition of the great vessels
Fibroelastosis of the left ventricle
Anomalous left coronary artery ("adult" type)
Fused mitral valves
Cleft mitral leaflet
Perforated mitral leaflet
Double orifice of the mitral valve
Anomalous insertion of chordae tendineae

are usually poorly developed children with a history of easy fatiguability and frequent respiratory infections. The auscultatory findings are similar in rheumatic and isolated congenital mitral regurgitation. Husson and his associates (1964) have suggested that marked posterior transmission of the systolic murmur is "diagnostic" of a congenital mitral lesion. In mitral regurgitation due to a defect in the anterior leaflet, the "jet stream" is directed against the atrial wall adjacent to the vertebral column and the systolic murmur is heard well posteriorly. However, wide transmission to the back is not uncommon in patients with severe rheumatic mitral regurgitation. The roentgenographic and electrocardiographic findings re-effect the severity and duration of the heart disease and the abnormalities are usually more marked, therefore, in children with congenital mitral valve defects. In general, the age of the child, long duration of heart disease, and severity of the mitral incompetence favor the diagnosis of a congenital defect.

The differential diagnosis of aortic regurgitation is less difficult because in children there are few nonrheumatic causes of this lesion. As previously emphasized, the murmur of aortic regurgitation can be easily missed during acute rheumatic carditis. It is not uncommon to encounter patients with aortic regurgitation who have either no history of rheumatic fever or an ill defined illness which may have been rheumatic fever. Congenital aortic insufficiency without other cardiac abnormalities has been reported, but it is extremely rare (Frahm et al., 1961). The diastolic murmurs of a patent ductus arteriosus, aortopulmonary window, and aortic regurgitation associated with a ventricular septal defect are not usually difficult to distinguish from rheumatic aortic regurgitation, since these defects have the distinctive features of a left to right shunt. A short diastolic murmur along the left sternal border can be heard in patients with severe anemia and in thyrotoxicosis. Aortic incompetence is common in patients with Marfan's syndrome but the classic features of the tall thin child with poor eyesight are easily recognized.

Sickle Cell Disease.   Cardiac enlargement, loud and changing heart murmurs, and electrocardiographic changes are common in children with sickle cell disease. Since these patients may also have fever, epistaxis, abdominal pain, and joint pains, their symptoms can be easily confused with acute rheumatic fever. The diagnosis can be made by the demonstration of red cell sickling and hemoglobin electrophoresis studies. The coexistence of sickle cell disease and rheumatic fever is rare (Uzsoy, 1963).

Differential Diagnosis of Chorea

The insidious onset of emotional changes, purposeless movements, and muscle weakness are characteristic of chorea. Early in the course of the illness, the only symptom may be a change in the child's behavior so that a functional disorder due to school or family conflicts is suspected. It is only when incoordination and random movements appear that the diagnosis becomes obvious.

Tics or habit spasms are sometimes confused with chorea. These conditions should not be difficult to distinguish. Habit spasms follow a set, repetitive pattern involving the same muscle groups; choreiform movements are ever changing. The fidgety, hyperactive movements of a child who cannot sit still are occasionally incorrectly attributed to chorea. These children may be emotionally disturbed but the movements are coordinated and there is no muscle weakness.

Choreiform movements may rarely be caused by organic central nervous system disease, congenital or acquired. Although it is usually not difficult to distinguish chorea from true athetosis, occasionally the random movements of the athetoid patient resemble chorea. Unlike Sydenham's chorea, however, the movements are not of recent onset and other signs of neurologic involvement are present.

Errors in Interpretation of Minor Manifestations

History. It is important to obtain a past history of rheumatic fever, but the evidence should be documented by a careful and detailed description of events, and past hospital records should be obtained whenever possible. Often a past history of rheumatic fever is accepted on the basis of inadequate information and is used to support a diagnosis of rheumatic fever in patients who do not fulfill the Jones criteria. Although a strong family history may add to the suspicion of rheumatic fever, such a history should not weigh the diagnosis unduly in children who do not meet the criteria.

Fever. Protracted low-grade fever in a child may lead to the suspicion of rheumatic fever, especially if it is accompanied by vague aches and pains and if the fever follows an upper respiratory infection. Often this "fever" is within the normal diurnal temperature variations and if the parents can be sufficiently reassured and persuaded to stop recording temperatures, a rapid cure frequently results. On the other hand, if fever has indeed been present for a protracted period, it is rarely due to rheumatic fever in the absence of other manifestations. The diagnosis of rheumatic fever should never be made on the basis of fever alone, merely because no other cause can be found.

Arthralgia. Arthralgia is a common and genuine rheumatic symptom. However the loose application of this term often leads to the overdiagnosis of rheumatic fever. All too often the term is employed to describe pain in muscle, bone, bursa, and tendon, above or below the joint, indeed, to limb pain of almost any kind. Such complaints occur frequently in childhood and are usually due to innocuous causes. The most common are so-called "growing pains" which can be easily differentiated

Table 12. Differences Between Joint Pains of Subacute Rheumatic Fever and Nonrheumatic Leg Pains*

Clinical Condition	Joint Pains of Subacute Rheumatic Fever	Nonrheumatic Leg Pains (Growing Pains)
Time of pain	During entire day. Disappears on getting warm in bed. Worse on first getting out of bed in morning.	At end of day or soon after falling asleep. Free of pain in morning.
Location of pain	In joints. Pain on motion. Child points out pain in joints. Involves joints in upper extremities. May cause limping.	In muscles of thighs and legs. No pain on motion. Child vague in pointing out site of pain. Pain in upper extremities unusual.
Other signs of rheumatic activity	Common—nosebleeds, fever, pallor, abdominal cramps, undernourishment, carditis.	Usually none.
Other findings in joints	Local heat, mild swelling, tenderness on pressure.	None.
Family history of rheumatic fever	Common.	Rare.
Significant laboratory findings	Sedimentation rate increased.	Sedimentation rate normal.

* Modified from Shapiro, J. J.: Mod. Conc. Cardiov. Dis. 24:295, 1955.

from rheumatic arthralgia (Table 12). Faulty arches and other abnormalities of the feet not infrequently contribute to recurrent leg pains. Muscle pains may be associated with or follow respiratory infections and if accompanied by protracted low-grade fever and an innocent heart murmur, an incorrect diagnosis of rheumatic fever is often entertained. Arthralgic pains may occur following German measles. More serious ailments such as leukemia and sickle cell disease cause severe limb pain and may masquerade as rheumatic fever. Although every child with true arthralgia should be thoroughly investigated, the possibility that the arthralgia is due to rheumatic fever can often be excluded by a careful history and physical examination.

Abdominal Pain. Rheumatic abdominal pain can be exceedingly difficult to distinguish from early acute appendicitis, particularly since the abdominal symptoms frequently precede other rheumatic manifestations. In contrast to appendicitis, the pain is usually generalized and is less likely to become localized to the right lower quadrant. The temperature is usually higher in acute rheumatic fever than in appendicitis. The white blood count is elevated in both conditions. The sedimentation rate is often significantly elevated in rheumatic fever and normal or slightly elevated in acute appendicitis. Whenever the diagnosis is in doubt, a sedimentation rate determination may be very helpful. If the diagnosis remains in doubt, it is better to advise operation than to risk rupture of the appendix and peritonitis.

Misinterpretation of Laboratory Findings

Streptococcal Antibodies. Patients with illnesses which simulate rheumatic fever may by chance have an elevated streptococcal antibody titer, particularly when there is a high incidence of streptococcal disease in the community. Although an elevated streptococcal antibody titer is proof of a recent infection with these organisms, it is *not* in itself sufficient to establish the diagnosis of rheumatic fever. Streptococcal antibody levels tend to be higher in rheumatic patients than in children with uncomplicated streptococcal infections, but the magnitude of the titer is not diagnostic of rheumatic fever. It must therefore be emphasized that immunologic evidence of streptococcal infection must always be correlated with the clinical findings before a conclusion is reached.

Acute Phase Reactants. The acute phase reactants are abnormal in a wide variety of inflammatory conditions and neither an elevated ESR nor a positive CRP is specific for rheumatic fever. Since the CRP is a serologic determination and is the newer of the two commonly used tests, it is sometimes mistakenly thought to be more specific for rheumatic fever than the ESR. Both are good screening procedures for inflammatory processes but any acute or chronic infection of a nonrheumatic nature may cause these tests to be abnormal. Determinations of acute phase reactants and streptococcal antibody titers must be evaluated in conjunction with a careful history and the physical findings.

Chapter Ten

TREATMENT OF RHEUMATIC
FEVER AND CHOREA

In any disease in which the pathogenesis has not been completely elucidated, treatment remains unsatisfactory. The only specific therapy in rheumatic fever which has been suggested is based on the knowledge that group A streptococci play an essential role in this disease.

ANTIBACTERIAL AGENTS

Sulfonamides. Sulfanilamide was the first antibacterial agent shown to be active against group A streptococci. In 1938 Swift et al. and Massell and Jones treated patients with acute rheumatic fever with sulfanilamide. Both studies showed that this drug had no beneficial effect and often tended to exacerbate the symptoms. Sulfonamides are now never used for the treatment of acute rheumatic fever.

Penicillin. For many years it had been assumed that the action of streptococci in rheumatic fever must be indirect: the usual bacterial inflammatory reaction does not occur and streptococci cannot usually be demonstrated in the lesions. However, in 1939, findings of several English pathologists suggested that this assumption might need revision. Green (1939), Collis (1939), and Thomson and Innes (1940) reported independently that they had isolated group A streptococci from the valves of patients dying of acute rheumatic fever. Between 1939 and 1941 one attempt to confirm these observations was unsuccessful (Watson et al., 1961). Further bacteriologic studies of autopsy material have not been undertaken in recent years because the failure to isolate streptococci

96

might be attributed to the widespread use of antibiotics in rheumatic patients.

In 1944, penicillin was tried in patients with acute rheumatic fever. Watson et al. (1944) gave 975,000 to 3,470,000 units of penicillin either intramuscularly or intravenously over a 2 week period to 8 young adult males. Foster et al. (1944) treated 38 young men for 5 days with a total of 1 million units given intramuscularly. Both these studies showed that penicillin in the dosage given had no effect on the clinical manifestations of rheumatic fever.

In 1950, in the course of studies on the prevention of initial attacks of rheumatic fever, Rammelkamp and his co-workers (Denny et al., 1950) recorded observations which suggested that the persistence of streptococci might be the crucial factor in determining whether or not rheumatic fever developed and that the streptococci in rheumatic valves reported by the English pathologists might be the focus where these organisms persisted. It seemed possible, therefore, that rheumatic fever was a form of bacterial endocarditis. To test this hypothesis, Rammelkamp and his co-workers tried massive doses of penicillin in patients with acute rheumatic fever (Mortimer et al., 1959). Children with initial attacks of rheumatic fever were divided into two matched groups: one group was given a total of over 48 million units of penicillin over a 6 week period; the other received no antibacterial medication. There was no difference between the two groups in the clinical or laboratory response during the acute phase of the illness. At the end of 6 weeks, children in both groups received prophylactic penicillin for the prevention of streptococcal infections. A comparison of the cardiac status at the end of 1 year suggested that the incidence of heart disease in the treated group had been decreased. In the opinion of Stollerman (1960) and other observers (Yearbook of Pediatrics 1959-1960), the evidence presented by Mortimer and his associates was not conclusive. Furthermore, Carter et al. (1962) were unable to confirm the findings reported by Mortimer et al. (1959).

Recommended Antibiotic Therapy

Although penicillin does not exert a favorable effect on the acute manifestations of rheumatic fever, it is considered advisable to eliminate streptococci completely before a prophylactic regimen is started. Throat cultures for streptococci are frequently negative at the time the diagnosis of rheumatic fever is established. The failure to isolate these organisms may be due to the previous administration of antimicrobial agents, or to their spontaneous disappearance during the latent period between the antecedent pharyngitis and the onset of rheumatic symptoms. However, a negative throat culture does not exclude the possibility that streptococci may still be present in the pharyngeal tissues or tonsils. Therefore, every patient with acute rheumatic fever or chorea should receive penicillin in amounts to maintain therapeutic levels for 10 days. A single intramuscular injection of 600,000 to 900,000 units of benzathine penicillin G is satisfactory. If oral medication is preferred, 200,000 to 250,000 units of penicillin 4 times daily should be given for 10 days. If the patient is sensitive to penicillin, erythromycin may be used in a dosage of 250 mg. 4 times daily for 10 days. Because of the danger of contracting infections with other types of beta hemolytic streptococci while in the hospital or at home, the regimen chosen for continuous prophylaxis should be started immediately after the 10 day course of penicillin therapy is completed. An additional advantage is that while the patient is under close observation the prophylactic regimen can be changed if any untoward reactions occur.

SUPPRESSIVE AGENTS

The most commonly used drugs in the treatment of rheumatic fever are salicylates and steroids. Both drugs have been employed extensively but there are still many divergent opinions regarding their value. Claims have been made for both of these drugs at one time or another indicating that: (1) they reduce the severity of the attack and may therefore be life-saving, (2) they shorten the course of the illness, and (3) they minimize or prevent heart damage. Only the more important reports bearing on these three effects will be discussed.

Salicylates.   Maclagan in 1876 popularized the use of salicylates for the treatment of rheumatic fever. He tried the bark of willow belonging to the natural family of Salicaceae since he thought that "a remedy for that disease would most hopefully be looked for among the plants whose favorite habitat presented conditions analogous to those under which the rheumatic miasm seemed most to prevail."

More than 60 years ago, Lees (1903) suggested large doses of salicylates as a "specific" antirheumatic agent. In 1943 Coburn re-emphasized the importance of massive doses. In his opinion salicylate given intravenously to obtain levels of 35 to 50 mg. per 100 ml. was necessary to prevent heart disease. Several observers agreed that large doses were better than small (Taran and Jacobs, 1945; Manchester, 1946; Reid, 1948). However, the data presented did not establish the validity of this conclusion. Other investigators were not convinced of the superiority of massive doses (Keith and Ross, 1945; Jager and Alway, 1946; Watkinson, 1949). Toxic reactions were common with intravenous administration and two deaths were reported in children (Taran and Jacobs, 1945). At the present time salicylates are rarely given intravenously and massive doses are not recommended.

Despite the long history of salicylate therapy in rheumatic fever, few controlled prospective studies were published before 1950. Illingworth et al. (1954) reviewed 170 papers on the treatment of rheumatic fever with salicylates. The studies were often based on small numbers of patients of different ages with a variety of different rheumatic manifestations. Most of the data presented were contradictory and inconclusive. Concurrent observations on matched controls were rarely included. More recent studies comparing conventional doses of salicylates and bed rest alone showed that the acute manifestations of rheumatic fever such as fever and joint manifestations did subside more rapidly in the treated than in untreated groups (Illingworth et al., 1957; Bywaters and Thomas, 1961; Dorfman et al., 1961). However there was no evidence that salicylates shortened the period of rheumatic activity and follow-up observations on the incidence of residual heart disease did not indicate any significant differences in patients given salicylates as compared to those treated only with bed rest. Bywaters and Thomas (1961) reported that the cardiac status of some of their patients deteriorated during salicylate therapy and suggested that salicylates may have precipitated congestive failure. Studies by Alexander and Smith (1962) support the conclusion that salicylates may be potentially dangerous in patients with active rheumatic carditis. These investigators showed that salicylates increase oxygen consumption and cardiac work. Further studies are needed to confirm these observations.

Although salicylates do not appear to prevent cardiac damage, they do have a dramatic effect on fever and joint inflammation. How salicylates act to reduce the symptoms and signs of inflammation remains unanswered. There is some evidence that salicylates diminish hyperemia and exudation by suppressing inflammatory substances which increase vascular permeability (Spector and Willoughby, 1963; Adams and Cobb, 1963; Collier, 1963).

Steroids. Hench and his co-workers (1949) were the first to treat acute rheumatic fever with cortisone. Although the clinical response of fever and arthritis was excellent, it was the impression of these investigators that the symptoms were merely suppressed and that the course of the disease was not shortened (Barnes et al., 1951). However, other observers were impressed with the effects of hormone therapy. It was shown experimentally that steroids decreased vascular permeability and diminished exudation and the migration of inflammatory cells (Thorn et al., 1953). It seemed possible that these effects on the inflammatory process might reduce the degree of scarring in the heart.

It soon became apparent that an extensive controlled study was needed to evaluate these new drugs. In 1950, the American Heart Association in cooperation with the Medical Research Council of Great Britain initiated a study for this purpose. Salicylates had been standard therapy for rheumatic fever for many years. It was therefore decided to compare the effect of hormone therapy (cortisone and ACTH) with aspirin to see if the new drugs represented a significant advance.

Cooperative Rheumatic Fever Study

The U.K. and U.S. Joint Study (1955) was designed to answer the following questions: (1) What is the relative effectiveness of ACTH, cortisone, and aspirin in altering the course of the acute disease, or in suppressing its clinical manifestations? (2) What is the relative effectiveness of these three agents in preventing rheumatic heart disease? The clinical trial was carefully planned to yield data suitable for statistical analysis. Prescribed dosages of each of the three drugs were given, and clinical and laboratory observations were made at specified intervals. All patients received penicillin to maintain therapeutic levels for 14 days to eradicate foci of streptococci, followed by oral sulfadiazine to prevent intercurrent streptococcal infections during the hospital stay and throughout the follow-up period. Only children under 16 years of age who met the modified Jones criteria (1955) for the diagnosis of rheumatic fever were included. Each of the three drugs was given for a total of 6 weeks followed by a 3 week observation period. Conventional doses of aspirin adjusted according to weight were employed. The same dosages of cortisone and of ACTH were used for all patients irrespective of age or weight: the total dosage of ACTH given intramuscularly was 1160 U.S.P. units; the total dosage of intramuscular cortisone 4050 mg.

It was found that hormone therapy resulted in more prompt control of certain acute manifestations, chiefly fever and arthritis, but there was a greater tendency for these manifestations to reappear following cessation of treatment. At the end of 1 year there was no significant difference among the three treatment groups in the incidence of heart disease. The data on 445 of the original group of 497 children were again analyzed after 5 years (U.K. and U.S. Joint Report, 1960) and the findings were entirely in accord with those reported after 1 year. Moreover it was apparent that irrespective of the therapy employed, the incidence of residual heart disease was directly related to the initial cardiac findings observed at the time of admission to the study (Table 13).

Other Studies

At the time the Cooperative Study was conducted, Harris and co-workers (1956) treated a smaller group of patients with similar doses of hormone therapy and compared the results obtained to a control group treated with bed rest alone. They did not find any significant effect on the cardiac findings in the hormone-treated group as compared with the

Table. 13. Prognosis in Relation to Cardiac Status at Start of Treatment*

Cardiac Status at Start of Treatment	No. of Cases Observed for 5 Years	Per Cent with No Murmur at 5 Years	No. of Deaths in 5 Years
No carditis	71	96	0
Questionable carditis	32	84	0
Apical systolic murmur, grade I only	39	82	0
Apical systolic murmur, grade II or III only	60	68	2
Apical systolic and apical mid-diastolic murmurs	44	48	1†
Basal diastolic with or without other murmurs	45 (15)‡	53 (27)‡	1
Failure and/or pericarditis	33	30	1
Pre-existing heart disease without failure and/or pericarditis	80	30	5§
Pre-existing heart disease with failure and/or pericarditis	22	0	6

* The combined results of all three treatment groups. Modified from U.K. and U.S. Joint Report: Circulation 22:503, 1960.
† Death from acute nephritis and uremia.
‡ Excluding one U.K. center.
§ Includes 1 death from acute intestinal obstruction.

controls either during the acute episode or 5 to 8 years later (Friedman et al., 1962).

Numerous reports have been published suggesting that the failure of these earlier studies to demonstrate the superiority of steroid over salicylate therapy or bed rest alone might have been related to the dosages used or the duration of treatment. Most of the studies which followed the Cooperative Study did not include observations on concurrent controls and frequently did not define either the initial cardiac findings or the comparability of patients allotted to the various treatment groups. However, a small number of controlled studies were done. Some of these papers are summarized in the following pages and the results of uncontrolled and controlled studies compared.

Large Doses of Steroids for Prolonged Periods: Uncontrolled Studies. Greenman and his co-workers (1953) were among the first to report good results with large doses of steroids. They treated a small series of patients who had carditis in their initial attacks with 300 mg. of cortisone daily for 6 to 8 weeks. The majority of these children recovered without residual heart disease. Done and his co-workers (1955) stressed the importance of individualizing steroid therapy. These observers varied the dosage of ACTH and of cortisone according to the weight of the patients and continued treatment until all signs of rheumatic activity subsided. After an average follow-up period of 3 years the incidence of heart disease in the hormone-treated groups was low compared to that of the patients treated with salicylates or bed rest. However, since all the patients in this study were not treated concurrently, the results could not be considered conclusive. Other investigators also reported a low incidence of residual heart disease in patients treated early in the course of their illness with moderately large amounts of steroids given for 10 to 12 weeks (Markowitz and Kuttner, 1955; Roy and Massell, 1956; Ferencz et al., 1959; Massell et al., 1961). Again, none of these studies included patients treated concurrently with salicylates or bed rest alone and no valid conclusions can be drawn from the results.

Large Doses of Steroids for Prolonged Periods: Controlled Studies. To determine whether large doses of steroids were indeed superior to salicylates, the pediatric cardiac services of eight hospitals situated in different cities agreed to pool suitable cases for a controlled study (Combined Rheumatic Fever Study Group, 1960). Patients with their first attack of rheumatic fever, onset within 28 days, who had clinical signs of *moderate to severe carditis*, were divided into two groups on a blind random basis. Care was taken to exclude children with mild carditis since the majority of these patients recover completely regardless of which suppressive agent is used. To draw valid conclusions in the trial of two therapeutic agents in a disease as variable as rheumatic fever, it is essential that the patients assigned to each of the treatment groups are comparable in age, severity of the attack, and duration of illness before the institution of therapy. A comparison of the clinical data in both groups is shown in Table 14.

Twenty-nine patients allotted to the prednisone group received 3 grams of prednisone over a period of 12 weeks. Twenty-eight patients were assigned to the aspirin group. Four of these 28 children were changed to prednisone because in the opinion of the chief investigators their con-

Table 14. Large Doses of Steroids for 12 Weeks: Controlled Study[*] Comparison of Clinical Data in 57 Patients

	Prednisone	*Aspirin*
Number of Patients	29	28
Average age: years	10	8.7
Average length of interval before therapy: days	13	10
Apical systolic murmurs		
grade 2	7	6
grade 3	21	21
Mitral diastolic murmur	15	19
Aortic diastolic murmur	2	2
Cardiac enlargement	14	17
Pericarditis	1	3
Congestive heart failure	1	3

[*] From Combined Rheumatic Fever Study Group: New Eng. J. Med. 262:895, 1960.

Table 15. Large Doses of Steroids for 12 Weeks: Controlled Study*
Results of Treatment One Year After Completion of
Therapy in 55 Patients†

	Prednisone	Aspirin	Aspirin Changed to Prednisone
No evidence of heart disease	12	16	1
Rheumatic heart disease	16	7	3
Total number of patients	28	23	4

* From Combined Rheumatic Fever Study Group: New Eng. J. Med. 262:895, 1960.

† One patient died and one was lost to follow-up.

dition was considered to be critical. After 1 year 28 patients given prednisone and 27 who had received the prescribed aspirin dosage were available for comparison. The incidence of heart disease in the two groups was essentially the same (Table 15). No evidence was obtained to indicate that prednisone given in large doses for 12 weeks was more effective than aspirin for the prevention of residual rheumatic heart disease. Of the 4 patients changed from aspirin to prednisone 1 died; after 1 year 2 have heart disease and 1 has a normal heart. In this study the patients were allotted to the two treatment groups on a random *single* blind basis. The medical staff therefore was aware of which drug the patient was receiving. The decision to change these 4 children from aspirin to prednisone may have been influenced by bias. In the opinion of most clinicians steroids control the acute exudative phase of rheumatic myocarditis more promptly than salicylates. However, to prove conclusively that steroids are indeed life-saving, a study of an adequate number of critically ill patients treated on a random *double* blind basis is essential.

In contrast to the results obtained in the Combined Rheumatic Fever Study (1960), Dorfman and his co-workers (1961) reported that large doses of steroids continued for 12 weeks were more effective than salicylates in the prevention of heart disease. However, in their total group of 85 patients with carditis in the initial attack, 26 (30 per cent) had minimal carditis manifested by systolic murmurs, grade 1/6 at the onset. It was shown in U.K. and U.S. Joint Report (1960) and in a subsequent study by the Combined Rheumatic Fever Study Group (1965) that patients with mild carditis, irrespective of the therapy employed, rarely develop residual rheumatic heart disease. It seems probable, therefore, that the inclusion of mild cases of carditis in the study by Dorfman and his associates might explain the difference between their findings and those of the first Combined Rheumatic Fever Study Group (1960).

Short-term Intensive Steroid Therapy: Uncontrolled Studies.   Wilson (1960) is the only observer who has claimed that steroids usually terminate rheumatic activity and prevent heart disease. In a series of papers

Table 16. Short-term Intensive Steroid Therapy: Controlled Study[*]
Comparison of Clinical Data in 73 Patients

	Prednisone	Aspirin
Number of Patients	34	39
Average age: years	8.1	8.7
Average length of interval before therapy:		
days	10.0	8.2
Apical systolic murmurs		
grade 2	10	14
grade 3	20	24
Aortic diastolic murmurs	5	3
Cardiac enlargement	15	24
Pericarditis	1	1
Congestive heart failure	2	9

[*] From Combined Rheumatic Fever Study Group: New Eng. J. Med. 272:63, 1965.

beginning in 1953, Wilson and her co-workers (1953; 1956; 1959; 1962) have reported that with large doses of steroids (100 to 160 mg. prednisone daily) given for 1 or 2 weeks, the majority of children recover without cardiac damage. None of these studies, however, included concurrent observations on patients treated with salicylates.

Short-term Intensive Steroid Therapy: Controlled Studies. In view of the favorable results reported by Wilson and her associates, the Combined Rheumatic Fever Study Group (1965) undertook a second study in which short-term intensive steroid therapy was compared with aspirin. Seventy-three patients with moderate to severe acute carditis in their first rheumatic attack were allotted to the two treatment groups on a random basis. Only children aged 14 years or younger, whose first rheumatic manifestation had occurred within 21 days of onset of therapy were admitted to the study. Prednisone, 3 mg. per pound of body weight per day, was given for 1 or 2 weeks. Aspirin, 50 mg. (¾ grain) per pound of body weight daily, was given for 6 weeks and then reduced to 25 mg. (½ grain) per pound per day for 2 additional weeks. A comparison of the clinical data in both treatment groups is shown in Table 16. The two groups were comparable, although a larger number of patients in the aspirin group had cardiac enlargement and congestive heart failure at the onset of therapy.

Thirty-four patients were allotted to the prednisone group. After a 7 day course, 15 of these 34 patients still showed signs indicative of persistent active carditis. These children were retreated with a second 7 day course of prednisone. After the second course signs of active carditis subsided in 7 but persisted in 8. After 1 year 19 of the 34 patients have heart disease (56 per cent). Thirty-nine patients were allotted to the

Table 17.   Short-term Intensive Steroid Therapy: Controlled Study*
Results of Treatment in 73 Patients One Year After
Completion of Therapy

		Prednisone	Aspirin	Aspirin Changed to Prednisone
Single Blind Study:† 39 patients	No heart disease	8	8	0
	Rheumatic heart disease	10	10§	3
Double Blind Study:‡ 34 patients	No heart disease	7	5	—
	Rheumatic heart disease	9	13	—

* Modified from Combined Rheumatic Fever Study Group: New Eng. J. Med. 272:63, 1965.
† Single blind: drug randomly allotted.
‡ Double blind: drug randomly allotted with medical staff unaware of which drug was being given.
§ One patient died.

aspirin group. Because of persistent signs of rheumatic activity 2 of the 39 children received a second course. In one of these patients, activity subsided. The other child developed congestive failure. Despite digitalis, diuretics, and transfusion, this patient died. After 1 year, excluding the child who died, 25 have heart disease, 26 of 39 (67 per cent). During the first part of the study, 3 patients were changed from aspirin to prednisone because the chief investigators considered their condition critical. In the second half of the study, to eliminate possible bias, medication was administered without the medical staff knowing which drug was being given (double blind) and no changes were made in the prescribed medication. These data are summarized in Table 17.

The difference in the incidence of cardiac sequelae between the two treatment groups was small and not statistically significant. Furthermore, in 8 patients rheumatic activity was not terminated despite two 7 day courses of intensive steroid therapy. Thus the results reported by Wilson and her co-workers were not confirmed.

Combined Steroids and Salicylates: Uncontrolled Studies. Gelli (1955) studied the effect of steroids combined with salicylates in 24 patients and reported good results. Fischel and his co-workers (1958) treated 41 patients with carditis in the initial or recurrent attack who ranged in age from 6 to 38 years. These observers recommended the use of steroids combined with salicylates and continuation of the salicylates when the steroids were withdrawn. With this regimen the severity of rebound phenomena appeared to be reduced. However, the authors stated that the number of cases were too few and in the absence of controls did not warrant definite conclusions on the effect of combined treatment on the incidence of heart disease. Illingworth and his co-workers (1957) compared six different therapeutic regimens among 200 children observed during a period of 9 years. The regimens employed were: (1) symptomatic only, 42 children; (2) salicylates in low dosage, 16 children; (3) salicylates in high dosage, 61 children; (4) steroids alone, 27 children; (5) steroids with salicylates in low dosage, 22 children; (6) steroids with salicylates in high dosage, 32 children. The patients were not allotted to the respective treatment groups on a blind, random basis and were not treated concurrently. The conclusion reached by these observers that the regimen of steroids combined with salicylates in high dosage is the most effective for the prevention of heart disease was not proved.

Summary. The studies that have been summarized indicate that salicylates and steroids are similar in several ways. Both are palliative and not curative. Neither drug appears to exert any effect on the unknown factor which initiates the rheumatic inflammatory process and there is no convincing evidence that either drug shortens the course of the illness. *In the opinion of most observers there has been no clear and consistent demonstration that cardiac damage is prevented or minimized by either salicylates or steroids even if used early in the course of the illness, in high or low dosages, or for long or short periods of time.* Both drugs are, however, effective anti-inflammatory agents for controlling the acute exudative manifestations of rheumatic fever. Clinical observations suggest that steroids may be more potent than salicylates and are more likely to produce a prompt subsidence of the acute manifestations. A short course of steroids is indicated, therefore, in severely ill patients in whom inflammatory edema of the myocardium may be life-threatening during the acute stage of the illness. Steroids offer no advantage over salicylates for milder cases. Rebounds are more frequent after the cessation of steroid therapy than following salicylates and prolonged administration may lead to serious toxic effects.

Recommended Suppressive Therapy

A general outline for the administration of steroids and salicylates is presented in this section. It represents a practical scheme of treatment derived from many years of clinical observation (Table 18). As new data become available, this schedule of therapy will undoubtedly need revision.

Polyarthritis with No or Minimal Carditis. Salicylates are the

Table 18. Recommended Suppressive Agents for Acute Rheumatic Fever

Clinical State:	Arthritis Only	Minimal Carditis	Definite Carditis No E.H.	Severe Carditis
Prednisone 1 mg./lb./day	0	0	7-10 days	2-4 weeks
Aspirin 50 mg./lb./day	1-2 weeks	2-4 weeks	6-8 weeks*	3-6 months†

* Aspirin therapy should be instituted at the time steroids are discontinued.
† Aspirin should be started 1 week before steroids are discontinued.

treatment of choice for patients with arthritis or mild carditis or both. Mild carditis is defined as follows: questionable cardiac enlargement, apical systolic murmurs of grade I to II, AV dissociation, prolonged PR interval. A dosage of 50 mg. of aspirin per pound of body weight administered in 6 divided doses over 24 hours will usually result in an adequate blood level (25 to 35 mg. per cent). In some cases it may be necessary to increase the dosage to 75 mg. per pound. After 1 or 2 weeks, if a satisfactory response has occurred, aspirin may be discontinued, and the patient observed for about 10 days. If there is no recurrence of symptoms, in many instances no further treatment is needed. However, in patients in whom arthralgia or fever persists or recurs, it is advisable to continue salicylates for 1 week after all clinical signs have subsided. It is not necessary to continue therapy if an elevated sedimentation rate is the only sign of rheumatic activity.

Children usually tolerate aspirin well. It may be taken with milk or after meals to decrease gastric acidity. Optimum therapeutic results are obtained with levels between 25 to 35 mg. per cent. Sodium bicarbonate increases the excretion of salicylates, and should not be given. The child must be watched for toxic reactions such as vomiting, tinnitus, and hyperpnea. If these symptoms occur, aspirin should be discontinued for a day or two, and resumed at a slightly lower dose. Most children prefer aspirin to sodium salicylate. Drugs such as phenylbutazone, gentisic acid, and other similar drugs have been tried, but offer no advantage over aspirin. Aminopyrine is highly effective in small doses, but should not be used because of the danger of agranulocytosis.

Carditis. Patients who have definite clinical signs of moderate to severe carditis of recent onset should be treated with steroids to bring the acute manifestations of the generalized inflammatory process under control as rapidly as possible. Prednisone has been widely employed and tends to cause fewer electrolyte disturbances than other steroids. A dose of 1 mg. per pound in 4 divided doses over a 24 hour period is usually sufficient for most patients. Steroids are continued until the patient's general condition has improved and the cardiac signs have stabilized. This response usually occurs within 7 to 10 days at which time the steroid can be discontinued without tapering and salicylates begun. Aspirin is continued until all clinical and laboratory signs of rheumatic activity have subsided.

Patients who have cardiac enlargement or heart failure at the onset of their illness should be continued on steroids for 2 to 4 weeks. When steroids are administered for more than 10 days, the dose must be tapered before discontinuing treatment. In such patients it is advisable to overlap steroid therapy with acetylsalicylic acid for 1 week before hormones are stopped in order to minimize rebound phenomena. Acetylsalicylic acid should then be continued until all signs of rheumatic activity have disappeared.

Short courses of steroid therapy are usually well tolerated. The well known complications of hypercorticism are minimal when therapy is limited to a 7 to 10 day period. Similarly, serious toxic effects, such as gastric ulcers or compression fractures of the spine, occur rarely, if at all, during short-term therapy. An unrecognized bacterial or any viral infection, particularly varicella, represents the most serious complications, and the physician must always be on the alert for such infections.

Rebound Phenomena

When suppressive therapy is reduced or discontinued in patients with acute rheumatic fever, clinical or laboratory signs of rheumatic activity may reappear. This reactivation is termed "rebound." Rebounds occur frequently when steroid medication is stopped or the dosage reduced. Signs of rheumatic activity may recur after treatment with salicylates, but they are usually milder and less common. The frequent occurrence of rebounds is additional evidence that suppressive agents do not "cure" the disease.

Rebounds may be mild or severe depending on the severity of the attack and on the point in the course of the rheumatic process that therapy is decreased or discontinued. Rebounds usually occur as the suppressive agent is tapered or within 2 weeks after cessation of treatment. Mild rebounds are characterized by fever, arthralgia, or mild arthritis. Murmurs which had disappeared may again become audible. The ESR is elevated and the CRP positive. In many instances mild rebounds are limited to abnormal laboratory findings. Severe rebounds are observed most frequently in children with established heart disease and cardiomegaly. Pericarditis, an increase in heart size, and congestive failure may occur. The severity of the disease during a rebound may be as great as or greater than at the start of treatment.

The mechanisms of the rebound phenomenon are poorly understood. It was formerly thought rebounds were due to adrenal-pituitary suppression. However, this would not account for rebounds following salicylates, since it has been shown that salicylates do not effect the adrenal-pituitary axis. The simplest explanation is that the rheumatic inflammatory process has not run its course and the premature withdrawal of the suppressive agent allows the resumption of the natural duration of the disease. Bywaters and Thomas (1961) found evidence in favor of this hypothesis since they found that fewer rebounds occurred after a 12 week course of steroids than after a 6 week course. On the other hand, Feinstein et al. (1961) found that the incidence of rebounds rose as the duration of steroid treatment increased. These observers suggested that suppressive therapy prevents "dispersion" of the rheumatic inflammatory process and that the "accumulated residual inflammation" appears in the form of a rebound.

Mild rebounds usually subside spontaneously in a few days and rarely require medication. If the rebound is severe, it is often necessary to reinstitute suppressive therapy. Salicylates should be used since a subsequent rebound is less likely after salicylates than after steroids. Severe rebounds can often be prevented or minimized in patients who are treated initially with steroids, if salicylates are given concurrently as steroids are being tapered. Salicylates should then be continued for several weeks after cessation of steroid therapy.

TREATMENT OF CHOREA

A large number of therapeutic agents and suppressive drugs (steroids and salicylates) as well as sedatives and tranquilizers have been used to treat chorea. None of these drugs has proven to be uniformly effective. In an illness such as chorea in which exacerbation and improvement may alternate spontaneously, the evaluation of any drug is difficult. Fortunately it is a self-limited disease and irrespective of therapy, the emotional and neuromuscular signs and symptoms subside in 2 to 3 months in the majority of patients.

General Measures. It is usually advisable to take the child out of school when the diagnosis of chorea has been established. In exceptionally mild cases, particularly during a relapse or at the onset of a recurrence, a brief attempt may be made to continue school attendance after the teacher has been made fully aware of the child's condition. For most patients, however, bed rest is indicated. If the chorea is severe, a change in environment may be beneficial, and hospitalization is therefore frequently better than home care. Whether at home or in the hospital, a private room with a quiet atmosphere is desirable. Precautions must be taken to prevent the patient from bruising himself and from falling out of bed. The bed should have high sides which have been thoroughly padded. If the chorea is very severe, some type of restraint may be necessary. Sympathetic nursing care is an important requisite since patients with chorea are embarrassed and frustrated by their awkwardness. Careful attention should be paid to maintenance of fluids and nutrition for those children who are unable to feed themselves.

Sedation sometimes decreases the severity of the movements. Phenobarbital is often satisfactory for this purpose. Therapy with tranquilizers is entirely on a trial and error basis since the superiority of any special one has not been established. Bromides and chloral hydrate are rarely used.

Antistreptococcal Treatment. Every patient with chorea should receive a 10 day course of penicillin therapy followed immediately by a prophylactic regimen to prevent streptococcal infections.

Suppressive Drugs. Steroids have been reported to be of value in the treatment of chorea (Schwartzman et al., 1953; Ainger et al., 1955; Fletcher, 1960). Others, however, have not confirmed these results (Aronson et al., 1951; Dixon and Bywaters, 1952; Glaser and Merritt, 1952). Variation from patient to patient is so marked that observations on matched cases are not possible and valid data on the efficacy of one type of therapy as compared to another are not available. In our own experience, steroids have not appeared to influence the symptoms or course of patients with chorea.

Suppressive drugs may be indicated in patients with chorea and signs of an active rheumatic inflammatory process. In these patients a satisfactory response can usually be obtained with salicylates.

TREATMENT OF CONGESTIVE HEART FAILURE

General Measures. Children in heart failure should be placed at complete bed rest. They should not be allowed to feed themselves until the signs of acute failure are brought under control. The pat.ent should be placed in the orthopneic position in a moist, cool, oxygen tent. Morphine in doses of 1 mg. per 10 pounds of body weight is indicated if the patient is apprehensive or restless. Sodium intake should be restricted and fluid intake reduced.

Suppressive Drugs. As noted, steroid therapy should be used in severely ill patients with rheumatic myocarditis of *recent* onset. In children who have been ill for many weeks with or without heart failure, the value of steroids is questionable. Taran et al. (1954) was not impressed with the results obtained with cortisone or ACTH in patients with protracted carditis. On the other hand, Czoniczer and his associates (1964) suggested that steroids were more effective than salicylates in controlling heart failure and reducing the mortality of chronically ill rheumatic patients. However, the significance of these data, obtained in retrospective studies, is difficult to interpret.

It is our impression that in children with chronic activity and congestive heart failure, strict adherence to bed rest, salt restriction, appropriate adjustment of digitalis dose, and the use of diuretics will often result in improvement. If all these measures fail, a short course of steroids may be tried.

Digitalis. If the decompensation is mild, the signs and symptoms can often be controlled with bed rest, oxygen, and steroids. However, if no improvement occurs within 24 hours or if severe failure is present at the outset, digitalis is indicated. In the past, digitalis was thought to be of little value in active rheumatic carditis and the margin between an effective dose and digitalis toxicity was considered narrow (Gold and DeGraff, 1929; Schwartz and Schwedel, 1930; Sutton and Wychoff, 1931).

At the present time, however, most observers agree that the judicious use of digitalis is indicated in heart failure associated with active rheumatic carditis. Feinstein and Arevelo (1964) did not find a higher incidence of toxicity in active carditis than in inactive rheumatic heart disease.

During the acute stage, digoxin is the preparation of choice. It is absorbed well and an effect can be demonstrated 4 hours after an oral dose. It is excreted rapidly and toxic manifestations disappear in 24 to 48 hours. The initial total oral digitalizing dose for children is 0.02 mg. per pound of body weight. This dose is lower than is customarily recommended for children but patients with active carditis are sometimes exquisitely sensitive to digitalis and it is wise, therefore, to use a low starting dose. If the drug is given parenterally, two-thirds of this amount is used. One-half the total dose is administered initially and the remainder given in 2 equally divided doses at 4 to 6 hour intervals. The pulse should be checked carefully and an electrocardiogram should be taken before the administration of each dose during the initial period of digitalization. If a therapeutic effect is not achieved following the calculated total digitalizing dose, and if there are no signs of digitalis toxicity, one-fourth of the total dose may be repeated. However, further increments should be given with great caution. It is often difficult to decide whether nausea and vomiting or electrocardiographic changes are due to heart failure or to digitalis toxicity. It is generally best to assume that arrhythmias or heart block which appear de novo are due to digitalis. The daily maintenance dose is approximately 25 per cent of the total digitalizing dose, administered daily in 2 equally divided doses.

Diuretics. Diuretics are rarely needed in children with heart failure early in their course of the first attack. They should be tried, however, if the response to other anticongestive measures is inadequate. In patients with recurrent carditis superimposed on previous heart disease, diuretics are often needed. Mercurials are effective for short term use. Meralluride (Mercuhydrin) and Mercaptomerin (Thiomerin) are the preparations of choice. The average dose for children is 0.5 ml. every 2 to 3 days. Chlorothiazide (Diuril) is preferred for long-term use. An average oral dose for children is 250 mg. 2 to 3 times daily. Potassium intake should be increased when chlorothiazide is administered for long periods.

BED REST AND AMBULATION

Restriction of physical activity until the rheumatic process became quiescent was a time-honored method of treatment. It was based on the assumption that a relationship existed between the work load of the inflamed heart and the degree of residual scarring. Support for this concept came not from scientific proof but from clinical experience. Many observers noted that children with unrecognized active disease, who have been ambulatory for several weeks prior to hospitalization, often develop cardiac damage. Whether this is due to the physical activity or to other factors is not known.

The need for prolonged periods of bed rest has been questioned recently. This is not surprising in view of the present trend toward early ambulation in many conditions including tuberculosis and nephritis. It does seem reasonable that ambulation can be carried out more rapidly than was the custom in the past. Rheumatic fever is becoming a milder disease and the incidence of residual heart damage has declined. However, the speed of ambulation should be varied according to the severity and the course of the rheumatic attack (Table 19).

Table 19.   General Guide for Bed Rest and Ambulation in
Patients with Acute Rheumatic Fever

Clinical State:	Arthritis	Minimal Carditis	Definite Carditis No E.H.	Severe Carditis
Bed rest	1-2 weeks	2-4 weeks	2-3 months	3-6 months
Modified activity	2-6 weeks	2 months	3 months	6-12 months
Full activity	After 6 weeks	After 3 months	After 6 months	Individualize

Polyarthritis.   In patients with polyarthritis without carditis, prolonged bed rest is not necessary. The fever and joint symptoms are usually brought under control rapidly following treatment with salicylates. At the end of the first week, the CRP has usually become negative and the ESR has begun to decline. At this time the patient may be allowed bathroom privileges and physical activities increased gradually over the next 2 weeks even though the sedimentation rate may still be somewhat elevated. If no rebound occurs, the patient may be allowed to return to school. However, full physical activities, especially competitive sports, should not be resumed for another month. During this entire period the cardiac findings should be rechecked at frequent intervals to be sure that they have remained normal.

Carditis.   Several investigators have reported studies in which rheumatic fever patients with carditis have been allowed out of bed rapidly without apparent deleterious effects (Gibson and Fisher, 1958; Lendrum et al., 1959). These studies do not include suitable concurrent controls, and the incidence of residual heart disease was low, suggesting that the patients studied had mild carditis.

Children with signs of minimal cardiac involvement should be kept in bed long enough to ascertain that there is no increase in cardiac abnormalities. This is usually apparent in 2 to 4 weeks. If there is no evidence of progressive cardiac involvement, ambulation is begun and physical activity is increased gradually over a period of from 4 to 6 weeks. No matter how mild the carditis, it seems advisable to delay the return to school for at least 2 months from the time of onset. Thereafter no restrictions are necessary.

Patients with definite myocarditis and valvulitis are treated more cautiously even in the absence of cardiac enlargement. Patients should be kept in bed until: (1) the intensity of the heart murmurs has diminished or has become stabilized, (2) heart sounds are of good quality, (3) sleeping pulse is normal, and (4) the CRP is negative and the ESR decreasing. Improvement usually occurs after 2 to 3 months of bed rest. Physical activities should be increased by progressive stages over the next month. The child is permitted first to have bathroom privileges. This is followed by sitting in a wheelchair for increasing periods of time. During this stage he is allowed to participate in quiet recreational activities. Toward the end of the month he is allowed to walk about freely in preparation for discharge. If his physical findings remain stable, he is allowed to return to school. However, excessive physical activities should be avoided for another 2 months. This regimen may be considered too conservative by proponents of rapid ambulation. However, it is our strong conviction that patients with myocarditis should be managed cautiously since cardiac enlargement, heart failure, and even sudden death may occur occasionally in these children when they are permitted to become ambulant too rapidly.

Even more conservative management is essential for patients with definite cardiac enlargement with or without congestive failure. Complete bed rest should be maintained, if necessary with the aid of sedatives. Children with congestive failure should not be allowed to feed themselves. Bed rest is continued until (1) heart failure is controlled, (2) heart size has decreased or become stabilized, (3) sleeping pulse is below 100 per minute, (4) the hematocrit is rising or normal and the CRP is negative, and (5) there is a true weight gain. Convalescence may often take 6 months or longer. In a small percentage of cases signs of active myocarditis may persist beyond this period (Taranta et al., 1962). During this prolonged period of convalescence, quiet occupational and recreational therapy should be carried out and the patient's school lessons continued. Physical activities are introduced gradually, guided by heart size and pulse rate. About 30 per cent of these children recover completely and can lead unrestricted lives. The remainder need a planned program of physical activity consistent with their cardiac reserve.

PHYSICAL ACTIVITIES AFTER RECOVERY

The physician's recommendations in regard to physical activities after recovery should take into consideration the severity of the attack, the extent of residual heart disease, the symptoms and temperament of the patient, and the attitudes of the parents.

No Heart Disease.   Children who recover from an attack of rheumatic fever without cardiac damage do not need any restriction of their physical activities and should lead entirely normal lives. After the convalescent period, during the course of an unhurried and thorough discussion, the physician should make it clear to the parents that the child has recovered completely. Overprotective parents often do not heed this advice and it should be re-emphasized, therefore, at future visits. Occasionally school authorities will also indiscriminately restrict all patients with a past history of rheumatic fever. It is tragic to see children who have become emotionally disturbed because they have been unnecessarily excluded from normal activities.

Valvular Disease without Enlargement.   Patients who are left with valvular damage with no or minimal cardiac enlargement pose more problems than the group with completely normal cardiac findings. Many physicians restrict these patients from all competitive sports and other activities conducive to overexertion in spite of the fact that the prognosis in patients without cardiac enlargement is generally good. In approximately 25 per cent of the patients with mitral regurgitation who remain free of recurrences, the murmur will disappear in 5 years. Furthermore, studies in adults suggest that, barring recurrent rheumatic fever and bacterial endocarditis, the prognosis is excellent in the majority of patients with "pure" mitral regurgitation (Jhaveri et al., 1960). Moreover, there is no evidence that restriction of physical activity improves the prognosis of these patients (Feinstein et al., 1962). Provided these children are under medical supervision and adherence to the prophylactic regimen is maintained, it is probably not necessary to restrict physical activity.

Valvular Disease with Enlargement.   Patients with a severe initial episode of rheumatic fever or with recurrent attacks often have residual valvular disease with some degree of persistent cardiac enlargement. Although their convalescence may be prolonged, the majority eventually tolerate ordinary physical activities well. These children should, however, be advised to avoid excessive fatigue, which is likely to be incurred in competitive sports. On the other hand, recreational activities requiring only moderate physical exertion should be encouraged to enable the patient to lead as normal a life as possible.

Chapter Eleven

CLINICAL COURSE AND PROGNOSIS

CLINICAL COURSE

The clinical course of rheumatic fever varies greatly. Most observers agree, however, that the *average* duration of an untreated attack is 3 months (Massell, 1958; Dorfman et al., 1961). If severe carditis is present, the duration is often longer than 3 months and signs of an active rheumatic process may continue for as long as 6 months. In a very small percentage of patients, less than 5 per cent, rheumatic fever remains active for more than 6 months. The latter cases are classified as "chronic" rheumatic fever.

Rheumatic fever is considered active if any *one* of the following findings is present: (1) joint symptoms, (2) new significant murmurs, (3) increasing heart size, (4) congestive heart failure in the absence of old valvular disease, (5) subcutaneous nodules, (6) rectal temperature over 100.4° F. for at least 3 consecutive days, (7) a sleeping pulse rate of more than 100 per minute, and (8) a positive C-reactive protein. An elevated sedimentation rate which persists for more than 6 months after the onset of the attack is not considered a sign of activity in the absence of other findings.

Polyarthritis

The joint symptoms may persist from a few days to several weeks if anti-inflammatory treatment is withheld. In a group of 16 untreated patients reported by Dorfman et al. (1961), the joints returned to normal

Table 20.   Incidence of Development of Significant Murmurs at Various
Intervals After the Onset of Initial Attacks of Rheumatic Fever*

Duration of Illness (Days)	Per Cent of Patients with Carditis Developing Heart Murmurs
1- 7	76.0
8-14	6.8
15-28	3.9
29-42	2.9
43-91	3.9
More than 91	6.8

* Modified from Massell et al.: Amer. J. Cardiol. *1*:436, 1958.

in 1 week in 8. In the remaining 8 patients joint involvement persisted for
7 to 59 days. It is not uncommon for the sedimentation rate to remain
elevated for several weeks after the joint symptoms subside. The natural
course of the illness is rarely observed in patients with polyarthritis since
the administration of suppressive drugs usually affords dramatic relief of
joint pain within 72 hours. Symptoms may return after anti-inflammatory
medication is discontinued when the attack has not yet run its course.
Suppressive drugs do not shorten the total duration of the attack.

Patients with rheumatic arthritis who have no abnormal cardiac findings within the first few weeks of their illness usually do not develop
carditis. Massell et al. (1958) studied the relationship of the development
of significant heart murmurs to the duration of illness (Table 20). Among
the children who developed carditis, a heart murmur was already present
during the first week of illness in 76 per cent. Seven per cent developed
a heart murmur during the second week and in 4 per cent the murmur
appeared between the second and fourth week of illness. Seven per cent
developed a murmur between the first and third month after onset.

Carditis

In patients with acute rheumatic fever with minimal signs of carditis
(poor quality heart sounds, borderline cardiac enlargement, electrocardiographic changes), the abnormal cardiac findings usually disappear
rapidly and the course of the illness is similar to that of the group with
"pure" polyarthritis.

In children with moderate or severe carditis, on the other hand, the
duration of rheumatic activity is longer than in patients without cardiac
involvement. Feinstein and Spagnuolo (1961) reported that the mean
duration of rheumatic activity in an untreated group of children with
carditis was 108 ± 34 days as compared to 79 ± 33 days in patients
without cardiac involvement (Table 21). In patients with carditis, after
the acute clinical symptoms subside, low-grade fever and tachycardia

Table 21.   Total Duration of Rheumatic Activity in 265 Patients
with Rheumatic Fever*

Cardiac Status	Anti-inflammatory Medication		Untreated	
	No. of Pts.	Mean Duration (Days)	No. of Pts.	Mean Duration (Days)
No carditis	95	91 ± 27	19	79 ± 33
Carditis	136	126 ± 70	15	108 ± 34

* Modified from Feinstein and Spagnuolo: J.A.M.A. 175:1117, 1961.

often continue, cardiac enlargement may persist, and new murmurs appear. Congestive heart failure may occur at any time while the rheumatic process is still active. It is not uncommon for the signs of active disease to persist for 3 to 6 months after the onset of illness.

The influence of anti-inflammatory drugs on the duration of rheumatic activity has been studied by Feinstein and Spagnuolo (1961). These investigators reported that the mean duration of activity was shorter in patients if no suppressive drugs were given (Table 21). They also studied the duration of rheumatic activity in patients with carditis in whom clinical rebounds occurred shortly after withdrawal of anti-inflammatory therapy. Data on the effect of treating rebounds on the duration of rheumatic activity are presented in Table 22. If the rebounds were allowed to subside without medication, the mean duration was essentially the same as in the untreated patients (Table 21). On the other hand, if the rebounds were retreated with suppressive drugs, the mean duration was increased by 2 months (62 days) in children without carditis and by 3 months (94 days) in those with cardiac involvement. Suppressive therapy reduces the amount of inflammation to subclinical levels, but does not terminate the active process. If the anti-inflammatory medication is given for a period shorter than the time required for the spontaneous subsidence of the inflammation, rebounds occur. If the rebound is treated with suppressive therapy, the inflammation is again suppressed, but its complete subsidence is delayed for a period of time

Table 22.   Total Duration of Rheumatic Activity in 64 Patients with
Post-therapeutic Clinical Rebounds*

Cardiac Status	Clinical Rebounds Treated With Suppressive Agents		Rebounds not Treated	
	No. of Pts.	Mean Duration (Days)	No. of Pts.	Mean Duration (Days)
No carditis	7	141	11	79
Carditis	26	206	20	112

* Adapted from Feinstein and Spagnuolo: J.A.M.A. 175:1117, 1961.

longer than that required for the spontaneous subsidence of the original inflammation (Feinstein and Spagnuolo, 1961).

"CHRONIC" RHEUMATIC FEVER

The majority of attacks of rheumatic fever are self-limited, and the reappearance of acute manifestations is due to a recurrence of the disease following an intercurrent streptococcal infection. As noted earlier, however, in a small proportion of patients the activity of rheumatic process becomes chronic, lasting more than 6 months. Taranta et al. (1962) reported 40 such cases among 1169 consecutive admissions to Irvington House, an incidence of 3 per cent. In 7 of these 40 children, chronic rheumatic activity developed following the initial attack of rheumatic fever. The remaining 33 patients had had one or more previous rheumatic episodes, indicating that the frequency of chronic rheumatic fever is greater in patients with recurrent attacks. Thirteen of 40 patients died within 8 months to 5½ years from the beginning of the "chronic" attack. Autopsies were obtained on 11 of these 13 children. All had congestive failure during the last 3 months of life. Four had auricular fibrillation and 3, fresh endocarditis. Seven of the 11 had positive acute phase reactants.

PROGNOSIS

The joint manifestations of rheumatic fever always subside completely without residua no matter how extensive and severe the arthritis. Likewise, despite prolonged and repeated attacks of chorea, no known impairment of the nervous system occurs. It is only in the heart that irreversible lesions may occur. The chief concern of the physician treating children with acute rheumatic fever, therefore, is to determine whether or not the heart is affected. Carditis still occurs in 40 to 50 per cent of initial attacks (Combined Rheumatic Fever Study Group, 1965). If signs of cardiac involvement are present, what is the likelihood that the patient will be left with residual rheumatic heart disease?

Relationship of Severity of Carditis to
Residual Rheumatic Heart Disease

It was clearly demonstrated in the U.K. and U.S. Joint Report (1960) that the more severe the cardiac involvement at the time the patient is first seen, the greater the incidence of residual rheumatic heart disease. In 103

Table 23. Prognosis in Relation to Cardiac Status at the
Start of Treatment*

Cardiac Status at Start of Treatment	Per Cent with Heart Disease after 5 Yrs.	No. of Deaths from Rheumatic Fever in 5 Yrs.
No or questionable carditis	8	0
Apical systolic, grade I	18	0
Apical systolic, grade II or III	32	2
Apical systolic and diastolic	52	0
Basal diastolic	47	1
Failure and/or pericarditis	70	1
Pre-existing heart disease	76	10

* Modified from U.K. and U.S. Joint Report: Circulation 22:503, 1960.

patients with no or questionable carditis, 95 (92 per cent) had no clinical evidence of rheumatic heart disease after 5 years, irrespective of whether ACTH, cortisone, or aspirin had been given. In a recent study (Combined Rheumatic Fever Study Group, 1965) among 87 patients with acute rheumatic polyarthritis, 20 children had signs of mild or questionable carditis. After 1 year these 20 children have normal hearts. The prognosis is also excellent in patients whose abnormal cardiac findings are limited to prolongation of the PR interval. Mirowski and co-workers (1964) followed 37 patients with polyarthritis and first degree heart block and found no evidence of residual heart disease. In a study of 80 acute rheumatic subjects with a prolonged PR interval, only 2 had rheumatic heart disease after an 8 year follow-up (Feinstein et al., 1964).

In patients with unequivocal evidence of carditis, the incidence of residual heart disease increases progressively in proportion to the severity of the cardiac involvement (Table 23). In the U.K. and U.S. Joint Study (1960), 18 per cent of patients with a grade I systolic murmur had residual heart disease. The percentage increased to 32 per cent in patients with a grade II or III apical systolic murmur, to 52 per cent in children with apical systolic and diastolic murmurs, and to 70 per cent in the group with congestive heart failure or pericarditis or both. The findings of the Combined Rheumatic Fever Study Group (1965) are similar (Table 24). In 73 children with moderate or severe carditis, 11 had con-

Table 24. Prognosis in Rheumatic Subjects with Congestive Heart
Failure and/or Cardiomegaly*

	No. Pts.	One Year Follow-up	
		Normal Heart	Heart Disease
Congestive failure	11	2	9
Cardiomegaly	30	9	21
	41	11	30 (73%)

* Combined Rheumatic Fever Study Group: New Eng. J. Med. 272:63, 1965.

gestive failure and 30 had cardiomegaly at the time of admission to the study. After 1 year 30 of these 41 patients (73 per cent) had heart disease. Both of these studies show that the patient's prognosis is directly related to the degree of *myocarditis*, manifested by cardiomegaly or heart failure.

Relationship of Recurrences to Prognosis

Carditis is likely to recur in patients in whom cardiac involvement was present in the initial attack and each recurrence may lead to further cardiac damage. The chief reason that we see fewer children with severe rheumatic heart disease at the present time is that prophylactic measures for the prevention of streptococcal infections in known rheumatic subjects are effective in reducing the incidence of recurrences.

Kuttner and Mayer (1963) reported that among 64 children with carditis in the first attack, 42 (66 per cent) had carditis in the second attack. Feinstein et al. (1964) recorded observations on 32 recurrences among 22 patients with known carditis at the time of the initial attack. There was evidence of further cardiac involvement in 17 of the patients with recurrences and approximately 25 per cent of these children developed additional cardiac damage.

Patients without clinical evidence of carditis in their first attack are less likely to acquire carditis in subsequent attacks and often escape residual rheumatic heart disease. Feinstein et al. (1964) studied 12 recurrences among 177 patients without previous cardiac involvement and noted evidence of carditis in 2, both of whom recovered without residual heart disease. In the series reported by Kuttner and Mayer (1963), among 50 patients without carditis during the first attack, 13 developed cardiac involvement during the second attack. Although patients without detectable signs of cardiac involvement in the first attack do not invariably escape carditis in subsequent attacks, the prognosis in the majority of these children is excellent.

Regression of Heart Disease

Follow-up studies of a large series of patients show that after 10 years heart disease may disappear in a significant number of patients (Table 25). Massell et al. (1959) reported 245 patients with carditis followed for varying periods of time with a maximum of 9 years. In his series, evidence of heart disease disappeared in 26 per cent. These investigators found that the regression of abnormal cardiac findings was related to the length of illness prior to admission to the hospital. Regression occurred most frequently in patients admitted within 14 days of onset, and was much less common in those who had been ill for 6 weeks or more when first seen. These authors emphasized that regression of abnormal cardiac findings rarely occurred in patients who had had congestive fail-

Table 25. Regression of Heart Disease Following
Acute Rheumatic Carditis

Study	No. of Pts. with Heart Disease	Length of Follow-up (Yrs.)	Cardiac Status at Follow-up	
			Normal Heart	Rheumatic Heart Disease
Ash (1948)	318	10	29 (9.4%)	289
Bland and Jones (1951)	653	10	76 (11%)	577
Massell et al. (1959)	245	9	65 (26.8%)	180
Feinstein et al. (1964)	188	8	45 (24%)	143

ure or pericarditis, cardiomegaly, aortic diastolic or mitral diastolic murmurs, or loud apical systolic murmurs.

Feinstein et al. (1964) also reported the disappearance of heart disease in a series of patients followed for almost 8 years. These investigators analyzed their data in relation to the murmurs present at the time that the patients were admitted to the study. In 61 patients with mitral insufficiency the systolic murmur disappeared in 23 children (38 per cent). In contrast to children with apical systolic murmurs only, heart disease persisted in 72 per cent of patients with diastolic murmurs, either mitral or aortic. Regression occurred most frequently in patients without cardiomegaly: in 36 children who had no cardiac enlargement evidence of heart disease disappeared in 19 (53 per cent). These investigators emphasize other important prognostic factors: (1) Cardiac lesions regress less frequently in patients who have had more than one attack of rheumatic fever. (2) The persistence of cardiac lesions is correlated more closely with cardiomegaly than with the extent of the valvular involvement. (3) Pericarditis in the absence of other evidence of severe carditis does not indicate an unfavorable prognosis.

Delayed Appearance of Heart Disease

As has been noted, new evidence of heart disease may occur in patients following recurrent attacks of rheumatic fever. Older studies suggested that heart disease developed not uncommonly in rheumatic subjects long after the initial attack of rheumatic fever in the absence of overt recurrences (Bland and Jones, 1951). In many of these patients it was assumed that a smoldering inflammatory process continued for years. More recent observations suggest that although chronically active carditis with progressive heart disease may occur, it is uncommon (Taranta et al., 1962). There is evidence to indicate that new or additional heart disease rarely develops in patients who receive antistreptococcal prophylaxis. In a series of 249 patients with no clinical heart disease following the first attack, only 3 developed heart disease subsequently (Feinstein et al., 1964). Progressive cardiomegaly may occur in children with valvular lesions due to hemodynamic factors. Children with mitral disease may ultimately develop mitral stenosis, but careful follow-up studies indicate that this lesion rarely if ever developed de novo (U.K. and U.S. Joint Report, 1960; Feinstein et al., 1964).

Deaths

It is well known that the death rate from acute rheumatic fever has declined markedly. In 1960 there was 0.4 death per 100,000 inhabitants due to acute rheumatic fever as compared to a rate of 16.8 in 1910 (Table 3). Childhood deaths from chronic rheumatic heart disease have also decreased. In one series there were 14 deaths among 426 rheumatic children followed for a period of 5 years (U.K. and U.S. Joint Report, 1960). In a group of 441 children and adolescents followed for an average of 8 years, 12 deaths were reported by Feinstein et al. (1964). Five of these 12 patients died following only a single attack of rheumatic fever. Among 304 patients observed at The House of the Good Samaritan, there were 5 deaths (Massell et al., 1958). On the basis of these studies, the case fatality rate for acute rheumatic fever and rheumatic heart disease in children ranges between 1.6 and 3.3 per cent.

Chapter Twelve

RHEUMATIC FEVER

RECURRENCES

One of the most striking characteristics of rheumatic fever is its tendency to recur. Prior to the introduction of preventive measures, from 60 to 75 per cent of patients with an initial attack of rheumatic fever had one or more recurrences (Roth et al., 1937).

PREDISPOSING FACTORS

Streptococcal Infections

A preceding streptococcal infection can be demonstrated in virtually every recurrence of rheumatic fever. The attack rate following such infections is much higher in a rheumatic than in a nonrheumatic population. In a carefully documented study in a convalescent home for rheumatic children, 14 recurrences were noted following 81 streptococcal infections, a recurrence rate of 16 per cent (Kuttner and Krumwiede, 1941). Wood et al. (1964) recorded 47 recurrences following 285 streptococcal infections in a long-term study of ambulatory rheumatic subjects. They found that although the recurrence rate was higher in patients with symptomatic sore throats, in many instances children with few or no symptoms of streptococcal infection also developed recurrences. They also showed that recurrence rates were related to the magnitude of immune response elicited by the antecedent streptococcal infection. On the other hand, recurrences could not be correlated with the pre-infection antibody titer nor with the number of previous streptococcal infections prior to the one which precipitated the rheumatic attack.

123

Interval Since Previous Attack

The recurrence rate is highest during the first 3 years following an initial attack. Roth et al. (1937) reported that of 488 patients with their first rheumatic episode, 73 per cent had a recurrence within 3 years. Marienfeld et al. (1964) studied the risk of second attacks in three age groups: 5 to 9, 10 to 14, and 15 years and over. The attack rate in all three age groups was greatest 1 year after the initial attack and decreased significantly within 3 years. Taranta and co-workers (1964) found that the number of recurrences per streptococcal infection dropped from 23 to 11 per cent as the interval since the preceding rheumatic attack increased (Table 26).

Table 26. Ratio of Rheumatic Recurrences to Streptococcal Infections According to Time Elapsed Since Onset of the Last Rheumatic Attack[*]

Interval Since Onset Last Attack (Months)	Ratio and Percentage of Recurrences to Infections
6-23	17/73 (23%)
24-41	16/94 (17%)
42-59	9/70 (13%)
60+	5/47 (11%)

[*] Modified from Taranta et al.: Ann. Intern. Med. *60:*(Pt. II) 58, 1964. The numerator is the number of recurrences and the denominator the number of streptococcal infections.

Previous Heart Disease

Susceptibility to recurrences is related to the presence and degree of heart disease. Taranta and co-workers (1964) have shown that the recurrence rate is greater in patients with heart disease and cardiomegaly than in patients with heart disease and no cardiac enlargement (Table 27).

Table 27. Ratio of Rheumatic Recurrence to Streptococcal Infections According to the Cardiac Status of the Patients Before the Infections[*]

Cardiac Status Before Infection	Ratio and Percentage of Recurrences to Infections
No heart disease	18/189 (10%)
Heart disease with no or slight cardiomegaly	20/74 (27%)
Heart disease with marked cardiomegaly	9/21 (43%)

[*] Modified from Taranta et al.: Ann. Intern. Med. *60:*(Pt. II) 58, 1964. The numerator is the number of recurrences and the denominator the number of streptococcal infections.

Age

The younger the child at the time of the initial attack, the greater the likelihood of recurrences. Carditis is often the presenting manifestation in children under 6 years of age and in these patients repeated attacks of carditis may occur before puberty. The incidence of recurrences usually diminishes after puberty. The decline with age is related to several factors. In civilian populations, adolescents and adults have fewer streptococcal infections than children, probably because of decreased exposure to infection. The recurrence rate per streptococcal infection is also lower in adolescents than in children (Table 28). Furthermore, as

Table 28. Percentage of Recurrences per Streptococcal Infection According to the Age of the Patient*

Age Group	Patient-years	% Recurrences per Strep. Infection
Children	338	14.8
Adolescents	530	6.5
Adults	225	4.5

* Modified from Stollerman, G. H.: J.A.M.A. 177:823, 1961.

an individual gets older the interval between attacks becomes longer and, as has been noted, the recurrence rate decreases as this interval lengthens. However, if heart disease is present, the decline in recurrence rate in older individuals is less marked.

Number of Preceding Attacks

The risk of recurrences increases with the number of previous attacks (Table 29). This is true in patients with and without heart disease, although patients with cardiac damage have a greater tendency to develop recurrences.

Thus, recurrences are more common when the initial attack strikes early in life, and when this attack includes carditis; they are more apt to

Table 29. Ratio of Rheumatic Recurrences to Streptococcal Infections According to Number of Previous Attacks of Rheumatic Fever*

No. Previous Attacks	Ratio and Percentage of Recurrences to Infections
1	20/185 (11%)
2	16/66 (24%)
3+	11/34 (32%)

* Modified from Taranta et al.: Ann. Intern. Med. 60: (Pt. II) 58, 1964. The numerator is the number of recurrences and the denominator the number of streptococcal infections.

occur soon after the prior attack than later, and are more frequent in childhood than in adult life; and finally, the risk of recurrence rises in proportion to the number of previous recurrences.

CLINICAL FEATURES

The signs and symptoms associated with recurrences are similar to those observed in the initial attack. The clinical and laboratory findings of active rheumatic fever have been described previously (Chapters 6 and 7). However, certain aspects of recurrences deserve special emphasis. They are: (1) mimetic clinical features, (2) problems in diagnosis, and (3) effect on the heart.

Mimetic Features of Rheumatic Recurrences

It was noted in many of the early studies that the same major clinical manifestations observed in the initial rheumatic episode usually recurred in subsequent attacks (Roth et al., 1937; Wilson and Lubschez, 1944; Bland and Jones, 1951). More recent surveys using uniform diagnostic criteria have confirmed and extended these observations. Feinstein and Spagnuolo (1960) reviewed the clinical features of 161 patients who had had 311 recurrences and noted the mimetic features of recurrences. One or more recurrences were observed in 90 patients who had cardiac involvement in the first attack. In 54, new signs of carditis developed. On the other hand, of 71 patients with normal cardiac findings during the first rheumatic episode, only 10 had carditis in a subsequent attack. These investigators thought it probable that in the latter group significant murmurs were present in the first attack and had been overlooked.

Kuttner and Mayer (1963) analyzed the cardiac findings during first and second attacks in 119 patients (Table 30). Fifty of 119 patients had no cardiac involvement during the first attack and of these, 13 had clinical evidence of carditis during the second attack. Among the 64 cases with cardiac involvement initially, evidence of new carditis occurred in 42 patients. These observers concluded that although rheumatic manifestations are often mimetic, in some instances the pattern varies.

Diagnosis

The diagnostic criteria are essentially the same for primary and recurrent attacks. It is sometimes difficult, however, to differentiate the onset of a recurrence from various nonrheumatic signs and symptoms. Rheumatic children are under continuous observation and frequently

Table 30. Cardiac Findings During First and Second
Attacks in 119 Patients*

1st Attack	2d Attack
64 cases of carditis	42 cases of carditis (65.6%) 6 cases of ? carditis (9.4%) 16 cases of no carditis (25%)
Total	64
5 cases of ? carditis	3 cases of carditis 1 case of ? carditis 1 case of no carditis
Total	5
50 cases of no carditis	13 cases of carditis (26%) 4 cases of ? carditis (8%) 33 cases of no carditis (66%)
Total	50
Total 119	119

* From Kuttner and Mayer: New Eng. J. Med. 268:1259, 1963.

have various complaints and signs which must be carefully evaluated. Perhaps the most common are fever and muscle and joint pains associated with viral infections. It is not uncommon for older children to complain of chest pain, palpitations, and even shortness of breath and yet have no evidence of heart disease. Peculiar movements due to either hyperactivity or habit spasms may simulate chorea. Suspicious complaints should not be disregarded since the early manifestations of active rheumatic fever or chorea may be extremely subtle. The laboratory findings can be of considerable help in distinguishing false alarms from true recurrent attacks. A rise in the ASO titer should always alert the physician for a possible recurrence, although the diagnosis should not be based solely on an elevated ASO titer. Tests for acute phase reactions are particularly valuable except in "pure" chorea. A recurrence rarely occurs without a definite significant rise in the erythrocyte sedimentation rate or a positive test for C-reactive protein. Both the ESR and CRP may be elevated in viral infections, but usually return to normal rapidly.

In patients with heart disease it is often difficult to establish the presence and degree of "new" carditis during a recurrence. Signs of pericarditis, involvement of an additional valve, the reappearance of a previous murmur, or marked increase in heart size are unequivocal signs of recurrent carditis. An increase in the intensity of murmurs previously present or slight changes in heart size are often more difficult to interpret. The appearance of congestive heart failure frequently indicates that active carditis is present, although in children with established valvular disease, cardiac decompensation may occur during the course of an intercurrent lower respiratory infection.

Effect of Recurrences on Cardiac Status

Rheumatic recurrences are less common and less likely to affect the heart in patients who escape cardiac damage in previous attacks. On the other hand, patients with heart disease not only have a greater number of recurrences but are also more prone to develop new carditis with each recurrence. The initial attack usually does not cause severe cardiac damage. In some an organic murmur may disappear only to return during the course of subsequent attacks. In 72 patients with recurrences reported by Feinstein and Spagnuolo (1962), a murmur reappeared in 9 and new additional murmurs were noted in 25. If significant heart disease persists following the first attack, recurrences not infrequently cause further cardiac damage. In a study reported by Guasch et al. (1962) the proportion of patients with heart disease increased with each recurrence from 67 to

Table 31. Relationship Between the Number of Attacks of Rheumatic Fever and the Severity of Valvular Heart Disease*

No. of Attacks	No. of Patients	No. with Heart Disease	No. with Severe Heart Disease
1	126	84 (67%)	6 (7%)
2	50	41 (82%)	6 (16%)
3	30	28 (93%)	9 (30%)

* Modified from Guasch et al.: Amer. J. Med. Sci. *244*:290, 1962.

93 per cent (Table 31). Furthermore the incidence of severe cardiac lesions increased from 7 to 30 per cent.

PREVENTION OF RHEUMATIC RECURRENCES

Once a patient has recovered from an attack of rheumatic fever, the physician's chief concern is the prevention of recurrences. No matter how mild the initial rheumatic episode, susceptibility to the disease is greatly increased and repeated attacks are likely to occur. As noted previously, both the incidence and severity of rheumatic fever have declined during the past 25 years. At the present time children with severe rheumatic heart disease are seen much less frequently than formerly. This decrease in the number of cases with debilitating rheumatic carditis cannot be attributed wholly to changes in the natural history of this disease but is due to a large extent to the introduction of prophylactic measures for the prevention of streptococcal infections and recurrences in known rheumatic subjects.

Methods of Prophylaxis

Sulfonamides

Sulfanilamide. Thomas and France (1939) and Coburn and Moore (1939) independently were the first to demonstrate that daily oral administration of small doses of this drug to rheumatic children prevented streptococcal infections and recurrences. These observations were quickly confirmed in numerous studies (Stowell and Button, 1941; Hansen et al., 1942; Chandler and Taussig, 1943; Kuttner and Reyersbach, 1943; Dodge et al., 1944; Feldt, 1944). A summary of the findings reported in these six studies shows a striking difference in the incidence of recurrences among the treated and untreated patients: Among 685 children serving as controls 137 (20 per cent) developed recurrences as compared to 12 recurrences (1.5 per cent) among 787 patients given small daily oral doses of sulfanilamide.

A small percentage of patients developed minor toxic reactions. However, 1 patient died of agranulocytosis. Since the advent of less toxic sulfonamides, sulfanilamide is no longer used.

Sulfadiazine. In World War II sulfadiazine was used for mass prophylaxis of military personnel. Holbrook (1944) reported that 1 gram of oral sulfadiazine daily prevented streptococcal pharyngitis and rheumatic fever. However after several months, sulfadiazine-resistant strains of group A streptococci, (types 17 and 19) began to cause pharyngitis followed by rheumatic fever (Epidemiology Unit, 1945; Damrosch, 1946). Mass prophylaxis with sulfadiazine was therefore discontinued (Coburn and Young, 1949).

Baldwin (1947) used sulfadiazine prophylaxis in a civilian population. In an outpatient cardiac clinic 102 children and adolescents were divided into two groups: one received 0.5 to 1.0 gram of oral sulfadiazine daily; the other group was untreated. During a 2 year period only 1 recurrence occurred in the treated as compared to 8 recurrences in the control group. No sulfadiazine-resistant strains of group A streptococci were isolated. None of the patients had renal complications and toxic reactions were uncommon.

An outbreak of scarlet fever due to sulfadiazine-resistant group A type 19 did occur in a small community in northern New York State (Johnson and Hartman, 1947). It was concluded that the strain had probably been introduced by contact with military personnel. During the past 18 years, sulfadiazine has been widely used. No other reports of sulfadiazine-resistant group A streptococci have been published.

Penicillin

As soon as penicillin became available, the possibility was explored that this antibiotic might prove superior to the sulfonamides for prophylaxis. Penicillin is bactericidal and the sulfonamides are bacteriostatic. The occurrence of penicillin-resistant group A streptococci had not been reported. The toxicity of this antibiotic was low and hypersensitivity reactions in children were infrequent.

Oral Penicillin. In 1947 penicillin lozenges were investigated as a means of preventing recurrences (Burke, 1947; Maliner and Amsterdam, 1947). In both these studies the number of patients studied was too small to warrant definite conclusions. In a second paper Maliner et al. (1949) found that penicillin lozenges containing 5000 units of penicillin given 3 times daily failed to produce demonstrable serum levels of penicillin. *Penicillin lozenges are not a satisfactory method for the administration of oral penicillin.*

Kohn et al. (1950) reported that in 64 rheumatic patients large doses of penicillin (1 million to 5 million units) given 5 days of each week, or for 1 week of each month, reduced the incidence of rheumatic recurrences as compared to comparable groups of untreated children. According to these observers, large doses of penicillin given intermittently were less likely to cause the emergence of penicillin-resistant strains of hemolytic streptococci than small doses given continuously (Milzer et al., 1948). Feinstein et al. (1964) studied intermittent as compared to continuous prophylactic oral penicillin and concluded that *continuous administration is essential for the prevention of rheumatic recurrences.*

Between 1950 and 1952 three controlled studies using oral penicillin for continuous prophylaxis in known rheumatic subjects were published. The dosages employed varied from 50,000 units given twice daily to 100,000 to 200,000 units once a day in a single dose (Brick et al., 1950; Evans, 1950; Gale et al., 1952). Only one of these reports was based on a sufficiently large number of children to warrant conclusions (Evans). Among 155 children in the penicillin group during a 2 year period there were no recurrences whereas among 145 patients serving as controls, 7 children had definite rheumatic attacks. In this study none of the group A streptococci isolated were penicillin-resistant. Prophylactic oral penicillin has been used extensively during the past 15 years. Penicillin-resistant strains of group A streptococci have not been encountered.

Oral penicillin is tolerated well by most children. Skin manifestations, chiefly urticaria, occur in less than 0.5 per cent of patients. If the penicillin is omitted for a few days, it can often be resumed without difficulty. More severe allergic reactions are rare, but when they occur, a different antistreptococcal drug should be used for prophylaxis.

Parenteral Penicillin. In 1952 Stollerman and Rusoff investigated a new repository penicillin preparation, benzathine penicillin G (Bicillin). After a single intramuscular injection of 1,200,000 units of benzathine penicillin G, adequate therapeutic levels were demonstrable in the majority of children for as long as 4 weeks. Monthly injections of this preparation proved effective in preventing streptococcal infections and recurrences of rheumatic fever. These findings were confirmed by other investigators (Diehl et al., 1954; Markowitz and Hemphill, 1955; Markowitz et al., 1957A).

The incidence of hypersensitivity reactions following the use of benzathine penicillin G in adults is 1 per cent (McFarland, 1958). Reactions are less common in children. Sherwood et al. (1957) reported that repeated injections of repository penicillin in army personnel caused no significant increase in reactions. The chief disadvantage of benzathine penicillin G is pain at the site of injection. Local soreness may last 2 or 3 days and interfere with school attendance. In many children local reactions become fairly well tolerated, but in some this preparation must be discontinued.

Comparison of Prophylactic Regimens

By 1952 three different antibacterial agents were available for the prevention of streptococcal upper respiratory infections and rheumatic recurrences in known rheumatic subjects: sulfonamide, oral penicillin, and parenteral penicillin. Different pediatric clinics used one or more of these drugs, but no conclusive evidence had been published to show which one was most effective for the prevention of rheumatic recurrences.

In 1954 a large-scale carefully controlled study was undertaken by Irvington House to compare the effectiveness of sulfadiazine, oral penicillin, and monthly injections of benzathine penicillin G. Four hundred and thirty-one known rheumatic patients were divided by a statistically controlled method of random selection into three comparable groups, each assigned to a different prophylactic agent. The results of this excellent

Table 32. Prophylaxis and Attack Rates of Streptococcal Infection and Rheumatic Fever Recurrences on 3 Prophylactic Regimens [*]

	Parenteral Benzathine Penicillin	Oral Penicillin	Oral Sulfadiazine	All Drugs
Number of patient-years	560	545	576	1,681
Number and rate of all streptococcal infections	34 (6.1)	113 (20.7)	138 (24.0)	284 (17.0)
Number and rate of all streptococcal infections, exclusive of carrier state	24 (4.3)	101 (18.5)	102 (17.7)	227 (13.5)
Number and rate of rheumatic recurrences	2 (0.4)	30 (5.5)	16 (2.8)	48 (2.9)

[*] From Wood et al.: Ann. Intern. Med. 60:(Pt. II) 31, 1964. Rates listed in parenthesis as number per 100 patient-years.

study are shown in Table 32. There were 1681 patient-years of observations: 560 on benzathine penicillin, 545 on oral penicillin, and 576 on sulfadiazine.

This study clearly shows that parenteral benzathine penicillin G is the most effective of these three prophylactic agents both for the prevention of streptococcal upper respiratory infections and for the prevention of rheumatic recurrences. The superiority of this regimen is probably related to several factors: (1) monthly visits to the clinic insure continuous prophylaxis; (2) absorption of the drug from an intramuscular depot is probably more complete than from the intestinal tract; (3) therapeutic levels of penicillin are sufficient to eradicate any intercurrent streptococci during 1 week of each 4 week interval.

No statistically significant difference between oral penicillin and oral sulfadiazine either in the prevention of streptococcal infections or of rheumatic recurrences was observed. No evidence was obtained to indicate that oral penicillin in a daily dose of 200,000 units was superior to 1 gram of oral sulfadiazine. In another study 1 gram of sulfadiazine daily was compared with oral penicillin 200,000 units given twice daily (Feinstein et al., 1964). Again sulfadiazine proved equally effective. Sulfonamide-resistant strains of group A streptococci were not encountered and in a civilian population this occurrence was considered unlikely. No major sensitivity reactions occurred during the 5 year period with oral or parenteral penicillin, or with sulfadiazine.

SELECTION OF PATIENTS

All children and adolescents who have a documented attack of rheumatic fever or chorea or who have rheumatic heart disease should be started on prophylactic treatment without delay. Many studies have shown that patients with polyarthritis or chorea without clinical signs of cardiac involvement often escape heart disease even if repeated attacks of polyarthritis or chorea occur (Feinstein and Spagnuolo, 1962). On the other hand, carditis occasionally does occur during second attacks in children who were considered to have normal hearts during their first attack (Kuttner and Mayer, 1963). Auscultatory techniques and x-ray examinations may not always be sufficiently sensitive to detect signs of minimal cardiac involvement. At the present time the majority of investigators hold the view that every rheumatic individual should be started on prophylaxis regardless of whether or not carditis is demonstrated.

Prophylaxis should be withheld in patients with ill defined illnesses which do not meet the criteria for a diagnosis of rheumatic fever. Unnecessary expense, exposure to drug reactions, and emotional trauma may result from the prolonged use of drugs in children incorrectly diagnosed as rheumatic subjects who do not need prophylaxis. There are occasions, however, when further observation is necessary before the diagnosis can be either established or excluded. In these patients prophylaxis should be instituted on a temporary basis until more thorough evaluation can be made.

CHOICE OF PROPHYLACTIC REGIMEN

Once it is established that a patient should receive prophylaxis, the physician must decide which regimen is most suitable for the patient and his family. The advantages and disadvantages of the three currently employed prophylactic regimens have been summarized by Stollerman (1960) (Table 33). The choice between oral and intramuscular medication should be based on several factors. Oral medication should be prescribed only if there is a reasonable assurance that the medication will

Table 33. Methods of Continuous Chemoprophylaxis of Streptococcal Infection*

	Sulfadiazine (Oral)	Penicillin (Oral)	Benzathine Penicillin (Respiratory)
Advantages	1. Easily administered 2. Well absorbed 3. Inexpensive 4. Established effectiveness	1. Bactericidal 2. Serious toxicity rare 3. No resistant streptococci	1. "Break" in prophylaxis less likely 2. Single dose usually eliminates carrier state 3. Economical 4. Close patient contact 5. Other advantages of penicillin (See Oral Penicillin)
Disadvantages	1. Frequent breaks in routine 2. Risk of serious toxicity 3. Resistant streptococci 4. Bacteriostatic	1. Frequent breaks in routine 2. Irregular absorption 3. Costly 4. Minimum effective dose not well established	1. Requires injection 2. Moderate local soreness
Recommended dose	1 g. per day	200,000-250,000 units once or twice daily	1,200,000 units intramuscularly once monthly
Toxicity	Skin eruptions—0.5% Blood reactions—0.01%	Urticaria angioneurosis "Serum type sickness" .02-.05% Anaphylaxis "Periarteritis" rare	Urticaria angioneurosis "Serum type sickness" 1-2% Anaphylaxis "Periarteritis"

* From Stollerman, G.: Acta Rheum. p. 45, 1960.

be taken regularly. It is often wise to give injections until a more thorough knowledge of the family is obtained. The maintenance of continuous prophylaxis is crucial in patients with established rheumatic heart disease and significant cardiomegaly. Repository penicillin should be recommended strongly to such patients and should be mandatory if it is obvious that lapses in oral medication are occurring.

Although a regimen of monthly injections of penicillin is the most effective, some children as well as their parents may object to injections and monthly visits to the clinic and may discontinue prophylaxis altogether. Oral medication is usually well accepted, and in families with adequate supervision the oral route is preferred. *There is no evidence that oral penicillin is better than sulfadiazine.* Oral penicillin has the disadvantage that it should be taken under fasting conditions (Markowitz and Kuttner, 1947). In children rushing off to school such timing is difficult. Sulfadiazine, on the other hand, can be taken after breakfast or at any time during the day.

DURATION OF PROPHYLAXIS

Most physicians agree that prophylaxis should be maintained for a minimal period of 5 years after an attack when the risk of recurrences is the greatest. How long to continue prophylaxis past puberty and into adult life is an unsettled question. Johnson et al. (1964) published data on 8 adolescents and 2 adults who developed rheumatic recurrences when prophylaxis was discontinued after 5 or more years. In the 8 adolescents the last rheumatic attack had occurred 6 to 9 years previously. In 1 adult the date of the previous attack was not known, but in the other the interval was 29 years. All of these 10 patients had preceding proven streptococcal infections. These observers concluded that although the frequency of both streptococcal infections and recurrences declines with age, nevertheless late recurrences may occur.

The problem of rheumatic recurrences in adults has also been studied by Mortimer and Rammelkamp (1956). These investigators noted 14 recurrences among 77 patients (18 per cent) observed following a streptococcal infection. In 10 of the 14 patients, 5 or more years had elapsed since the last rheumatic episode. The effect of antibiotic therapy for respiratory infections in patients with a past history of rheumatic fever was also studied by these investigators. Twelve per cent of a group of 139 patients developed either a definite or a possible recurrence despite antibiotic treatment of the group A streptococcal infection. These observers concluded that it is unwise to rely on antibiotic treatment of a streptococcal infection and that prophylaxis should be maintained indefinitely. Whether prolonged prophylaxis is needed for adults with normal hearts remains controversial. However, it is generally agreed that individuals with established heart disease, especially if accompanied by cardiomegaly, should receive life-long prophylaxis.

Prophylaxis Failures

Approximately 5 per cent of patients on oral prophylaxis (sulfadiazine or penicillin) and less than 1 per cent on parenteral penicillin develop recurrences. With oral prophylaxis, the major reason for failures is a lapse in taking the prescribed medication. In a study by Wood and associates (1964) the number of streptococcal infections and recurrences correlated directly with the dependability of the patient in taking the medication. Problems related to prophylaxis maintenance and suggested measures for improvement are reviewed elsewhere (page 180).

Streptococcal infections and recurrences occur in some patients in spite of regular prophylactic medication. In a study of an outbreak in a convalescent home, 11 of 33 rheumatic subjects developed streptococcal infections despite the supervised administration of 200,000 units of oral penicillin daily (Markowitz, 1957B). Virulent infections, a heavy inoculum of organisms, repeated exposures, and variations in absorption of penicillin probably all play a role. There is undoubtedly an irreducible minimal recurrence rate due to inherent deficiencies in preventive methods now available.

One of the major problems which plague secondary prevention programs is the number of drop-outs among adolescent patients. Marienfeld et al. (1964) studied the maintenance of prophylaxis in over 9000 college freshman who had had rheumatic fever. The survey was nationwide and included students from every state. Between 1935 and 1960 the number of individuals given prophylaxis following an initial attack increased every year. Following the publication by the American Heart Association of recommendations for prevention in 1953, the number of individuals placed on prophylaxis reached 80 per cent. Subsequently, however, with each passing year fewer students remained on prophylaxis so that eventually only 12.2 per cent of the 9044 students were taking medication. In the total group, 1433 individuals had had 2 or more recurrences. Despite this clear-cut evidence of the importance of prophylactic measures only 333 (23.6 per cent) of these 1433 students were on prophylaxis.

The tendency to discontinue prophylaxis occurs frequently, not only in private practice but also in special cardiac clinics in large hospitals, especially when adolescents are transferred from the pediatric to the adult cardiac service. Individuals with rheumatic heart disease often appear well and arouse little interest in the physician taking care of adult patients with overt symptoms. Prophylaxis is not stressed and the adolescent soon ceases to attend. A more thorough discussion of the drop-out problem is presented in Chapter 15.

TREATMENT OF STREPTOCOCCAL INFECTIONS IN RHEUMATIC PATIENTS

Adequate treatment of acute streptococcal infections with penicillin undoubtedly reduces the incidence of *initial* attacks of rheumatic fever (Chapter 14). On the other hand, it has not been established that similar treatment of streptococcal infections in rheumatic individuals not receiving prophylaxis, as well as those who "break through," will prevent recurrent attacks. In an outbreak of 11 cases of streptococcal pharyngitis in rheumatic children in a convalescent home, 4 children developed recurrences despite the prompt injection of 600,000 units of benzathine penicillin G at the time of the streptococcal infections (Markowitz, 1957B). It has been the experience of other observers that the use of much larger doses of penicillin than those described will not uniformly prevent recurrences in rheumatic subjects who develop streptococcal infections. Lim and Wilson (1960) have suggested that continuous prophylaxis is unnecessary and that recurrences can be prevented by prompt antibiotic treatment of every upper respiratory infection. However, in view of the experience noted, and since rheumatic recurrences frequently occur in patients without clinical signs of pharyngitis, *continuous prophylaxis is mandatory for every rheumatic individual.*

RELATIONSHIP OF TONSILLECTOMY TO STREPTOCOCCAL
ILLNESS AND RHEUMATIC FEVER

Studies by Holmes and Williams (1958) and Miller et al. (1958) based on bacteriologic data have suggested that streptococcal infections are less common in tonsillectomized individuals. A more recent epidemiologic study including serologic data has been reported by Chamovitz et al. (1960). These observers concluded that tonsillectomy (1) failed to reduce the risk of streptococcal infections, (2) did not alter the clinical course of the illness, and (3) failed to reduce the incidence of acute rheumatic fever or rheumatic valvulitis. Chamovitz and his associates have suggested that conclusions based only on bacteriologic data reported in previous studies may be misleading since streptococci tend to persist in individuals with tonsils. Although it remains unsettled whether or not streptococcal infections occur more frequently in patients with tonsils, there is no evidence to suggest that tonsillectomy reduces the incidence of initial or recurrent attacks of rheumatic fever (Wallace and Smith, 1936; Ash, 1938).

Chapter Thirteen

PREVENTION OF INITIAL

ATTACKS OF RHEUMATIC

FEVER (Primary Prevention)

One of the most significant advances in rheumatic fever during the past 15 years has been the demonstration that *initial* attacks of this disease may be prevented by adequate antibiotic therapy of the antecedent streptococcal infection. As noted previously (Chapter 2) this demonstration provided additional evidence of the importance of streptococcal infections in the etiology of rheumatic fever. The widespread use of antibiotics for respiratory infections has undoubtedly helped reduce the incidence of rheumatic fever, but the disease still occurs in circumstances in which it might have been prevented. Among 105 patients admitted in recent years to The House of the Good Samaritan with a first attack of rheumatic fever, not a single patient had received adequate therapy at the time of the antecedent streptococcal infection (Czoniczer et al., 1961). A similar experience was reported by Grossman and Stamler (1963).

At the present time acute rheumatic fever must be viewed as a potentially preventable complication of streptococcal infections, provided patients seek medical attention and receive adequate diagnosis and treatment. The studies on which the efficacy of primary prevention are based, the problems associated with the diagnosis of streptococcal infections, the recommended methods of treatment, and the present status of streptococcal immunization are discussed in this chapter.

PRIMARY PREVENTION STUDIES

The sulfonamides were the first antimicrobial agents proven effective in preventing streptococcal infections in known rheumatic subjects. However, the sulfonamides were found to be ineffective when given *after* the onset of the streptococcal infection (Coburn and Moore, 1939; Commission on Acute Respiratory Disease, 1945). These early observations were confirmed by the extensive studies of Morris and co-workers (1956). These investigators treated 261 patients with exudative pharyngitis due to group A streptococci with sulfadiazine. Forty-eight per cent still carried the organism 35 days after the onset of treatment. Pharyngitis recurred in 8 per cent and suppurative complications in 4 per cent. Of even greater significance was the fact that 14 patients (5.3 per cent) developed definite rheumatic fever and 6 additional patients had possible rheumatic fever. It was concluded from these studies that sulfonamides should not be used in the *treatment* of streptococcal infections.

The suggestion that penicillin treatment of streptococcal infections might prevent rheumatic fever was first made by Massell and co-workers (1948). Following their initial studies on a small group of patients, these investigators showed that a 10 day course of penicillin in 34 rheumatic subjects with streptococcal infections prevented recurrences in all but 2 patients, but 6 of 12 untreated children developed recurrences (Massell et al., 1951).

The studies by Massell were carried out in a rheumatic population. Subsequently, a group of workers led by Rammelkamp proved conclusively that primary attacks of rheumatic fever could be prevented in a *nonrheumatic* population. Rammelkamp and his associates were able to study large groups in military populations in whom streptococcal disease rates and the incidence of rheumatic fever were high. The military center was organized for the study of streptococcal infections: onset of the sore throat was known accurately, the diagnosis was confirmed by the isolation of streptococci from the pharynx, and careful follow-up studies were performed. Denny et al. (1950) showed that among 798 streptococcal infections treated with adequate amounts of penicillin only 2 definite cases of rheumatic fever occurred, in contrast to 17 cases of rheumatic fever among 804 untreated patients. These highly significant results were confirmed in a subsequent study (Wannamaker et al., 1951).

Persistence of the organisms following a streptococcal infection is the most significant single factor responsible for failure to prevent this complication (Catanzaro et al., 1958). Group A streptococci must be eradicated from the nasopharynx to reduce the incidence of rheumatic fever. Penicillin, a potent bactericidal agent, is the drug of choice. Administration in doses sufficient to maintain therapeutic blood levels for 10 days is essential to achieve a bacteriologic cure. Penicillin administered as late as 9 days after the onset of the streptococcal infection will still reduce the incidence of rheumatic fever (Catanzaro et al., 1954). Although penicillin is preferred, almost equally effective results have been obtained with tetracyclines (Hauser et al., 1953; Catanzaro et al., 1955). Effective therapeutic regimens are outlined later in this chapter.

All of these summarized studies on primary prevention were carried out in young adults during epidemics of scarlet fever or streptococcal pharyngitis with a high attack rate of rheumatic fever, 3 per cent. It has been difficult to perform comparable studies in children since endemic streptococcal infections are often mild and the incidence of rheumatic fever is low. The only controlled study in a childhood population has been reported by Siegel et al. (1961). Rheumatic fever did not occur among 519 adequately treated children with group A streptococcal infections, but 2 cases were observed among 532 untreated patients. Rheumatic fever has not been observed in several large series of children with streptococcal infections adequately treated with antibiotics (Breese and Disney, 1954; Stillerman and Bernstein, 1961; Markowitz, 1963). However, these studies did not include controls. The data available so far do not prove conclusively that first attacks of rheumatic fever are always preventable in a childhood population even if the recommended treatment is given. Most observers agree, however, that the concept of primary prevention proposed by Rammelkamp and his associates from studies in adults is applicable to children. As a result, considerable emphasis is being placed on the recognition and treatment of streptococcal infections as a means of reducing further the incidence of rheumatic fever.

DIAGNOSIS OF STREPTOCOCCAL INFECTIONS

Nasopharyngitis

Clinical Aspects. One of the obstacles to prevention of initial attacks of rheumatic fever is the difficulty of clinical diagnosis of streptococcal nasopharyngitis. The sudden onset of fever, pain on swallowing, beefy redness of the pharynx with exudate, and tender cervical nodes represents a characteristic syndrome of a streptococcal sore throat. A scarlatinal rash is diagnostic when it occurs but it is much less frequent than formerly. Scarlet fever is also less severe and at times the rash is less typical and difficult to distinguish from other exanthema. In children over 2 years of age, otitis media is often caused by group A streptococci, and such patients should receive the recommended therapy. The classic findings of streptococcal disease are more likely to be present during epidemics but occur only occasionally in patients with sporadic infections. The diagnosis is more difficult when tonsils are absent or when the patient is seen only once during the course of the illness, a fairly common occurrence at the present time. Several studies have shown that the physician can diagnose streptococcal infection clinically in 55 to 70 per cent of the cases (Breese and Disney, 1954; Siegel et al., 1961; Stillerman and Bernstein, 1961; Markowitz, 1963).

The chief problem is to distinguish mild streptococcal illnesses from viral infections of the upper respiratory tract. Conjunctivitis, coryza, hoarseness, and tracheitis are more likely to be due to a viral infection. However, it is not possible to distinguish bacterial from nonbacterial disease on the basis of pharyngeal redness alone. Indeed, even the occurrence of exudate, often considered the hallmark of a streptococcal infection, may not always be a reliable sign. Exudative pharyngitis has been described in association with adenovirus and Coxsackie virus infections (Shultz et al., 1960; Moffet et al., 1964). Shultz and his associates found that adenovirus, influenza, and undifferentiated respiratory disease could also each cause many of the other clinical features of streptococcal pharyngitis (Fig. 21). Similar findings are reported by Evans and Dick (1964).

Laboratory Aids.   The inability to recognize a significant percentage of streptococcal infections clinically has made the use of laboratory aids important. A white blood count may be helpful and a leukocytosis of

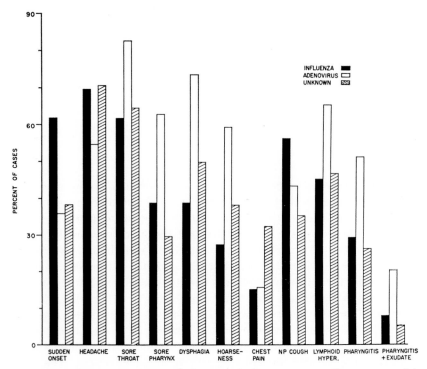

Figure 21. A comparison of the signs and symptoms in illnesses caused by influenza or adenovirus or of unknown etiology. (From Shultz et al.: J. Lab. Clin. Med. 55:504, 1960.)

more than 12,000 cells suggests a streptococcal rather than a viral infection. It is not, however, diagnostic. Bacteriologic confirmation by a culture of the pharynx is the most useful single laboratory procedure and should be employed in every patient in whom a streptococcal infection is suspected. Although the use of throat cultures has increased, experience suggests that there are still too many children with respiratory infections who consult physicians and do not benefit from modern diagnostic methods available for the identification of beta hemolytic streptococci. Practicing physicians who use throat cultures are generally able to prescribe antimicrobial agents more discriminately. They are better able to select the most effective antibiotic and prescribe sufficient dosage for the proper length of time.

Throat culture techniques are practical and bacteriologic interpretation is relatively simple. Bacteriologic studies can be readily accomplished in the physician's office by the use of inexpensive prepared media and an incubator which costs less than $75. Fluid media are not necessary. Sheep blood agar is superior for the recognition of beta hemolytic streptococci. Its chief advantage is the inhibition of the growth of colonies of hemophilus organisms which closely resemble those of beta hemolytic streptococci (Krumwiede and Kuttner, 1938). Sheep cell agar in disposable plastic plates is obtainable from many commercial laboratories.

The throat swab is inoculated directly on a small area on the blood agar plate. The inoculum is spread by streaking with a wire loop. When necessary, swabs well moistened with pharyngeal secretions may be kept for several hours at room temperature before inoculation. The plates can be read after overnight incubation at 37°C. Beta streptococci hemolyze the red blood cells in the medium completely and therefore are surrounded by a clear halo, in contrast to the greenish area visible around alpha streptococci. The large opaque colonies of hemolytic staphylococci also can be readily distinguished from streptococci.

It is advisable to estimate the number of colonies of beta hemolytic streptococci present. In patients with frank untreated infections numerous hemolytic colonies are usually obvious (Fig. 22). When there is a scant growth of hemolytic colonies, the question arises whether the beta hemolytic streptococci are the cause of the illness or represent a carrier state. In general, if more than 10 colonies are present, it is likely that the streptococci are playing an etiologic role. This assumption is probably not always correct and the physician must take into consideration the clinical as well as the bacteriologic findings.

In patients with clinical symptoms it is usually not necessary to group the streptococci because, almost without exception, such infections are due to group A streptococci. In special circumstances the bacitracin disc method for the identification of group A strains may be used (Maxted, 1953). A bacitracin disc, containing 0.02 unit of this antibiotic, placed on the agar plate will inhibit the growth of group A organisms and not that

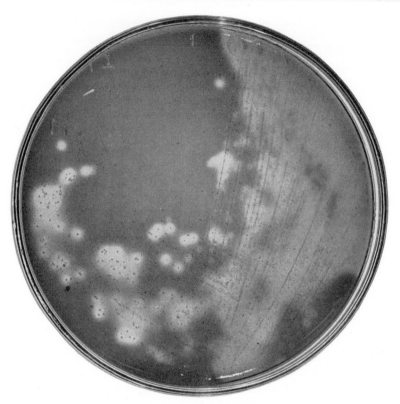

Figure 22.   Throat culture containing numerous colonies of beta hemolytic streptococci on sheep's blood agar medium in a disposable plastic plate.

of other groups (Fig. 23). This method is simple and is more than 90 per cent accurate (Streamer et al., 1962).

An increasing number of private laboratories and public health facilities are available for physicians who are unable or do not wish to perform their own bacteriology. Packets containing Dacron-tipped swabs can be mailed conveniently (Lattimer et al., 1963). Older methods for identifying group A streptococci are being replaced by immunofluorescent staining techniques (Warfield et al., 1961; Moody et al., 1963). The fluorescent antibody method gives more rapid results and identifies group A organisms directly. However it is not readily applicable for use in small clinical laboratories or in the physician's office.

Miscellaneous Streptococcal Infections

Streptococcal infections in children are not limited to the nasopharynx. Infection of the skin and vagina are not uncommon. It is generally believed that these infections are secondary to a nasopharyngitis but evidence for this assumption is inconclusive. Careful bacteriologic and

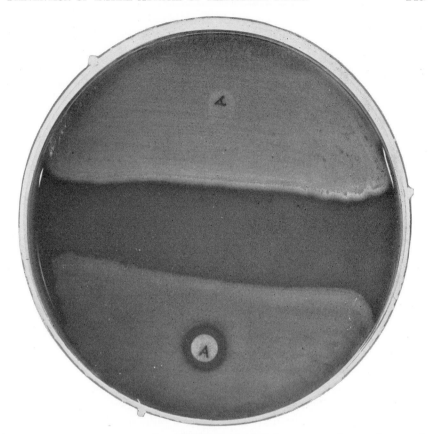

Figure 23. Bacitracin discs (labeled A) placed on pure cultures of group A and non-group A streptococci growing on a blood agar plate: growth of group A streptococci inhibited around the disc (lower half); the growth of non-group A streptococci was not affected.

immunologic studies have shown that evidence of a streptococcal infection can be demonstrated in approximately 40 per cent of children with impetigo (Markowitz et al., 1965). Although acute glomerulonephritis is frequently associated with streptococcal impetigo, skin infections rarely if ever precede either the initial or a recurrent attack of rheumatic fever. The reason that rheumatic fever does not follow streptococcal skin infections may be that these lesions are superficial and evoke little immune response (Markowitz et al., 1965).

TREATMENT OF STREPTOCOCCAL INFECTIONS

In ill, toxic children with symptoms and signs highly indicative of streptococcal pharyngitis (scarlatinal rash, acute adenitis, dysphagia, exudate), treatment should be begun immediately. In children with less characteristic findings, it is advisable to withhold treatment and await the results of the throat culture. Penicillin therapy is still effective despite a delay (Catanzaro et al., 1954). Once the diagnosis of a streptococcal pharyngitis has been established, the patient should be treated no matter how mild the clinical symptoms. Brumfitt et al. (1959) have introduced the concept of the "benign streptococcal sore throat" which is not followed by rheumatic fever. Rheumatic fever is more likely to follow an exudative pharyngitis than one with minimal symptoms (Siegel et al., 1961). However, in an outbreak of rheumatic fever described by Zimmerman et al. (1962), 8 of the 11 children had mild or subclinical streptococcal infections. Therefore it is still impossible to differentiate with any certainty the potentially dangerous from the benign streptococcal sore throat.

The principal aim of treatment is to eradicate streptococci from the nasopharynx. Clinical recovery alone is not sufficient. Persistence of the organisms is common following inadequate treatment and is the chief reason for failure to prevent rheumatic fever (Catanzaro et al., 1958). The properly selected antimicrobial agent must be administered in sufficient dosage to maintain therapeutic blood levels for 10 days. Penicillin, erythromycin, and tetracycline are satisfactory drugs. As noted previously, *sulfonamides should not be used for the treatment of streptococcal infections.*

Penicillin is the drug of choice. Group A streptococci have remained exquisitely sensitive to the bactericidal effect of penicillin. A number of preparations and therapeutic regimens are satisfactory. The most effective procedure is a single intramuscular injection of benzathine penicillin, 600,000 to 900,000 units in children and 1.2 million units in adolescents. With this therapy it is not essential for the patient to return to the physician or to remember to take daily oral medication. A single intramuscular injection will eliminate the streptococci in 95 per cent of the patients (Stollerman and Rusoff, 1952; Chamovitz et al., 1954). Benzathine penicillin may cause painful local reactions. An alternative regimen is 600,000 units of penicillin in oil with aluminum monostearate intramuscularly every third day for three doses. *A single injection of aqueous or procaine penicillin is inadequate* and repeated injections are generally impractical. Oral penicillin, 200 to 250,000 units 4 times daily, may be used. The oral preparations available are essentially similar (Breese and Disney, 1958). Penicillin G is the least expensive but should be taken under fasting conditions (Markowitz and Kuttner, 1947). The chief disadvantage of oral therapy is the common failure to complete the 10 day course, since the child is usually clinically well in 3 days and neither the parent nor the child understands why continued medication is necessary (Mohler et al., 1955; Bergman and Werner, 1963). Bacteriologic or clinical relapses occur in approximately 15 per cent of patients who have received the recommended therapy. Despite such therapy, symptoms may recur or cultures remain positive because of re-exposure to homologous streptococci through household contacts (Stillerman and Bernstein, 1964). Usually a second course of penicillin in a higher dose will eradicate the organisms. Treatment failures may be due to penicillinase-producing staphylococci which inactivate the bactericidal effects of penicillin (Frank and Miller, 1962; Simon and Sakai, 1963; Kundsin and Miller, 1964). Antistaphylococcal agents such as oxacillin may be effective in such cases (Simon and Sakai, 1963). However, oxacillin should be reserved for those patients in whom streptococci persist and the presence of penicillinase-producing staphylococci has been demonstrated.

Erythromycin is the drug of choice for patients who are sensitive to penicillin. A dose of 125 to 250 mg. 4 times daily for 10 days is effective. Tetracycline in a similar dosage and for an equal length of time may be used but it may be ineffective because an increasing number of tetracycline-resistant strains of group A streptococci are being encountered (Mogabgab and Pelon, 1958; Kuharic et al., 1960). Among 218 strains tested by Kuharic and his associates, 20 per cent were resistant to tetracycline. Tetracycline should not be used unless it is determined that the infecting organism is susceptible. Preparations containing combinations of antimicrobial agents offer no advantage in the treatment of patients with streptococcal infection and their use is not recommended.

Streptococcal Carriers

Streptococci may persist in the nasopharynx for long periods following an untreated infection. Krause and his co-workers (1962) were able to culture organisms from patients infected with an epidemic strain even after 3 to 5 months. These cultures usually contained fewer than 10 colonies and the streptococci often could not be typed. Krause and Rammelkamp (1962) showed a difference in the pathogenicity of group A streptococci isolated from a patient with pharyngitis during the acute and convalescent stages: the strain isolated during the acute stage was typable and caused infection when inoculated intranasally in monkeys; the strain obtained during the convalescent stage 20 weeks later could not be typed and failed to cause infection in monkeys.

The streptococcal carrier rate among children is high. Quinn and his associates (1957) found that cumulative carrier rate for the school year ranged from 57 per cent to 88 per cent among pupils in the third and fourth grade. Cornfeld et al. (1958) found that approximately half a school population of 1000 children had one or more positive cultures for beta hemolytic streptococci without clinical manifestations of infection. The majority of strains isolated in both studies were group A but a large percentage could not be typed.

Streptococcal carriage is not necessarily significant. In studies carried out in a convalescent home, Kuttner and Krumwiede (1944) found that "healthy carriers" do not commonly spread the organism to other individuals. A carrier is more likely to be dangerous if large numbers of organisms are present and if the strain is typable. The importance of nasal carriers in the spread of streptococci has been emphasized by Hamburger and his associates (1945). It is probably wise to limit the treatment of streptococcal carriers to those children who have had evidence of a recent infection, especially if they are members of a rheumatic family.

Mass culturing of school children has been undertaken in some areas as a method of controlling streptococcal infections in the community and reducing the incidence of rheumatic fever (Bunn and Bennett, 1955; Phibbs et al., 1958). However, a high proportion of children have been found to harbor beta hemolytic streptococci so that if all children who harbored streptococci were excluded from school, a great number would be absent. Furthermore, although penicillin treatment will reduce the number of carriers in some children, it is often exceedingly difficult to eradicate streptococci (Goerner et al., 1947). Many observers therefore feel that mass culturing of asymptomatic children is not a practical method for rheumatic fever prevention.

Prevention of Streptococcal Infection in
Nonrheumatic Individuals

Family Contacts. The management of other members of the family when the diagnosis of a streptococcal infection has been established poses special problems. Several studies have shown that there is a relatively high rate of spread of these organisms when there is an active infection in the household (Breese and Disney, 1956; James et al., 1960). Some physicians prescribe prophylactic doses of penicillin for several days for children and adults in contact with the infected individual. However, Breese and Disney noted that a number of the family contacts already have positive cultures at the time the diagnosis is made in the index case. Prophylactic doses of penicillin in these individuals are potentially dangerous since overt infection might be suppressed but the organisms not eradicated. James and his associates (1960) have recommended therapeutic doses of penicillin for a period of 10 days for all household contacts. However, this may be advisable only in families with a history of rheumatic fever. Ideally, throat cultures should be obtained and family members with significantly positive cultures be given a full course of treatment. The remainder of the family can then be placed on a prophylactic regimen. If cultures are not feasible, therapy can probably be safely withheld in a nonrheumatic family until signs and symptoms of illness appear.

Epidemics. Outbreaks of virulent streptococcal infections are common in military camps. They are often followed by a high attack rate of rheumatic fever and cause a significant loss in manpower. The control of streptococcal infections in the Armed Forces, therefore, is of considerable importance. A number of studies have demonstrated that mass prophylaxis can effectively abort epidemics and reduce the carrier rate (Wannamaker et al., 1953; Bernstein et al., 1954; Morris and Rammelkamp, 1957; Davis and Schmidt, 1957). The most effective agent is benzathine penicillin G, 900,000 to 1,200,000 units intramuscularly (Morris and Rammelkamp, 1957; Davis and Schmidt, 1957). Oral penicillin, 250,-000 units twice daily for 10 days, may be used (Bernstein et al., 1954). The use of mass prophylaxis in civilian populations has a more limited application but may be indicated at times in convalescent homes and boarding and public schools. Poskanzer and his associates (1956) showed that mass administration of oral penicillin to a school population during epidemics was practical and efficacious. These investigators found that 250,000 units twice daily for 10 days was effective but 250,000 units once daily was of little value. A case of rheumatic fever during a streptococcal outbreak in a school should alert health authorities to the possibility that a virulent "rheumatogenic" organism is present and that mass prophylaxis should be considered (Zimmerman et al., 1962).

STREPTOCOCCAL IMMUNIZATION

In any disease in which repeated attacks are common, active immunization would be preferable to antimicrobial prophylaxis. Although secondary prevention programs have been generally successful, failures due to omission of the drug are common. Even when the prescribed prophylactic regimen is conscientiously followed, breakthroughs occur. In primary prevention, penicillin is effective, but failures are inevitable because not infrequently the symptoms of streptococcal pharyngitis are trivial and transient, and the child does not receive medical attention. During the course of an extensive 2 year study of streptococcal infection and rheumatic fever in a village in the Netherlands, 4 cases of rheumatic fever were encountered and in each patient the rheumatic fever was preceded by subclinical pharyngitis not seen by physicians (Goslings et al., 1963). The limitations of both primary and secondary prophylaxis might be overcome if an effective biologic method of preventing streptococcal infections could be developed.

Antitoxin to the erythrogenic toxin of streptococci is readily produced in animals and develops in most patients following an attack of scarlet fever. Antitoxic immunity is life-long, but does not protect against infection with heterologous types of group A streptococci. Injection of erythrogenic toxin into rheumatic subjects, therefore, is of no value in preventing streptococcal infections and rheumatic recurrences (Coburn and Pauli, 1935). When intravenous injection of heat-killed streptococci was tried, severe reactions were encountered and no definite evidence was obtained to indicate that this type of treatment was beneficial (Wilson and Swift, 1931; Swift et al., 1931; Collis and Sheldon, 1932).

Immunity to streptococcal infections was better understood after it was shown by Lancefield that group A streptococci could be divided into specific types on the basis of distinct type-specific antigens, the M protein. Injection of these antigens into animals produced type-specific protective antibodies. Kuttner and Lenert (1944) demonstrated type-specific antibodies in children following streptococcal upper respiratory infections. These antibodies confer long-lasting immunity to the particular type causing the infection, but do not protect against infection with other types. Since there are 50 different types of group A streptococci, the problem of immunizing children appears formidable. However, only a relatively small number account for the majority of cases of streptococcal infection in a given community, so that a vaccine need not contain all known types (Smolens and Warner, 1952; Markowitz, 1963).

A second and more significant obstacle has been the difficulty in developing an antigenically potent vaccine of low toxicity. Killed whole streptococci cause severe reactions and an irregular antibody response (Rantz et al., 1949). With the development of methods to purify M protein, attempts were made to immunize with this partially purified antigen. Schmidt (1960) injected partially purified M proteins with adjuvant into a group of rheumatic children. The injections were well tolerated, but only 3 of 22 children developed bactericidal antibodies. Several groups of investigators have shown that because of the high M protein content, cell wall preparations are capable of stimulating the formation of type-specific antibodies in animals (Barkulis et al., 1958). Hayashi and Walsh (1961) successfully incorporated three different types in one vaccine. Potter et al. (1962), utilizing cell walls of type 5 and type 12, were able to boost or recall type-specific antibody in patients known to have been infected with the homologous types but were unable to produce a primary antibody response. Wolfe et al. (1963) have performed extensive studies with cell wall preparations as well as with M protein, with and without adjuvants. These investigators found that without adjuvants, these substances produced a secondary but not a primary immune response. However, when the M antigen was injected in mineral oil, 10 of 16 patients developed bactericidal antibodies. Although some of the patients developed sterile abscesses, no serious reactions were encountered. These findings are encouraging but it is obvious that the problem of an effective streptococcal vaccine is far from solved.

Chapter Fourteen

CHRONIC RHEUMATIC

HEART DISEASE

Acute carditis occurs in 40 to 50 per cent of children with their first attack of rheumatic fever. Permanent scarring of the myocardium or valves may result from the first rheumatic episode, but in most instances the first attack does not cause serious cardiac lesions. Irreversible damage develops most often in children who have had more than one attack. Chronic valvular deformities cause long-term hemodynamic disturbances and place an increased work load on the myocardium. Progressive cardiac enlargement and heart failure may ultimately develop, especially if there has been concomitant myocardial injury.

The mitral is the valve most frequently affected. It is involved three times more often than the aortic valve. Lesions limited to the aortic valve are less common but do occur. Not infrequently both the aortic and mitral valves are affected. In children, involvement of the tricuspid and pulmonic valves occurs rarely.

MITRAL REGURGITATION

Pathology

Mitral regurgitation may occur very early in the course of an acute attack, probably because of the edema and verrucae along the valve margins which prevent the cusps from sealing completely. If the valvulitis is mild, complete healing may occur and signs of mitral regurgitation may either disappear or be of no functional importance. However, if the inflammatory process is severe and involves the entire valve structure, permanent incompetence of the mitral valve results. The valve cusps

149

become thickened, rigid, and retracted, so that they do not meet to close the mitral orifice. Fusion and shortening of the chordae tendineae may restrict valve closure and dilatation of the mitral ring may aggravate the incompetence. As the left atrium and left ventricle enlarge, additional changes may occur. Edwards and Burchell (1958) have shown that the leaflets of the mitral valve are continuous with the endocardium of the left atrium and as this chamber dilates, the posterior leaflet is displaced away from the mitral orifice, thereby increasing mitral incompetence. Furthermore, as the left ventricle enlarges, the orientation of the papillary muscles and chordae tendineae changes, interfering with the apposition of the cusps (Levy and Edwards, 1962).

Hemodynamic Effects

The functional effects of mitral regurgitation depend on the degree of incompetence and the state of the myocardium. In childhood, regurgitation is often mild, and if the myocardium is in good condition, the hemodynamic disturbances are minimal. None of the cardiac chambers enlarge and the patient is asymptomatic. When there is marked incompetence, during systole a large amount of blood is ejected back into the left atrium since the pressure gradient between the left ventricle and left atrium is greater than that between the left ventricle and the aorta. The increase in the volume load causes dilation of the left atrium. As left atrial output increases, the diastolic volume in the left ventricle increases leading to dilation of this chamber. If the contractability of the myocardium is impaired, the left atrial pressure and left ventricular end diastolic pressure rise. This in turn increases pulmonary vascular resistance and burdens the right side of the heart.

Clinical Findings

Mild mitral regurgitation without cardiac enlargement is common in rheumatic children and an apical pansystolic murmur is the only abnormal clinical finding. In patients with moderate or severe mitral incompetence, the left precordium may become prominent and the apex is displaced downward and to the left. A left ventricular heave or lift may be noted and a systolic thrill may be palpated over the apical region. The first heart sound is normal or soft in intensity and is often incorporated in the systolic murmur. The second heart sound is frequently split, varying with respiration.

An apical systolic murmur is the hallmark of mitral regurgitation. Classically, it begins with the first heart sound and extends to the second sound (pansystolic), is blowing in quality, and is maximal over the apex with an intensity of grade 2/6 to 4/6. The murmur may be of the same intensity throughout systole, or it may be crescendo or decrescendo (Fig.

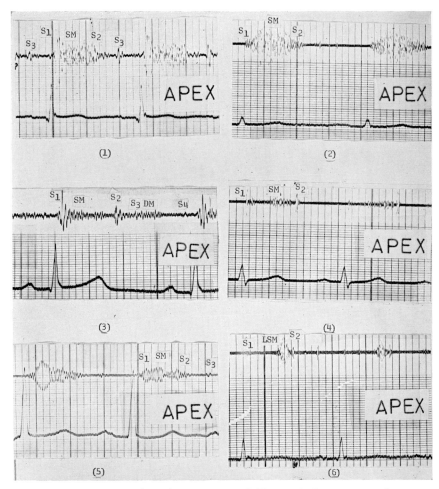

Figure 24. Types of systolic murmurs in children with rheumatic mitral regurgitation. (1) plateau, (2) midsystolic accentuation, (3) decrescendo, (4) crescendo, (5) inconstant pansystolic, (6) late systolic. S_1 = first heart sound. S_2 = second heart sound. S_3 = third heart sound. SM = systolic murmur. DM = diastolic murmur.

24). A mid or late systolic murmur, once thought to be innocent, can be caused by mitral incompetence (Barlow et al., 1963). The systolic murmur of mitral regurgitation is usually transmitted to the axilla and left scapula. However, it may be referred to the upper sternal area (Fig. 25). If the regurgitant jet is directed posteriorly and laterally against the atrial wall, the murmur is readily heard over the vertebral column (Perloff and Harvey, 1962). A third heart sound and a short mid-diastolic murmur are often audible when the mitral regurgitation is severe. The mid-diastolic murmur is generally attributed to rapid blood flow across the mitral opening and is similar to the Cary Coombs murmur heard during acute rheumatic fever. Recently, Nixon (1961) has proposed the view that third

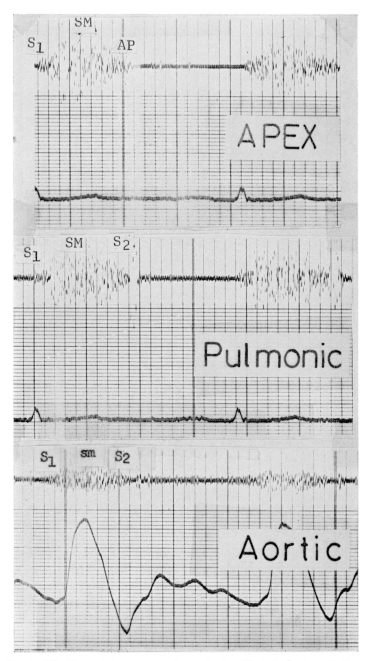

Figure 25. Pansysto.ic murmur in patient with mitral regurgitation. Note marked reference to pulmonic and aortic areas. S_1 = first heart sound. S_2 = second heart sound. SM = systolic murmur.

heart sound vibrations arise when the vigorous early diastolic elongation of the left ventricle tautens the mitral cusps and chordae. This also reduces the mitral orifice causing some obstruction to flow into the ventricles, and a mid-diastolic murmur results.

Radiologic Findings

The heart size varies with the degree and duration of mitral regurgitation. When enlargement of the left ventricle is present, transverse diameter of the heart in the posteroanterior view increases with elongation of left cardiac segment and displacement of the apex downward and to the left (Fig. 26).

In the pediatric age group, mitral regurgitation is the most common cause of left atrial enlargement and this chamber may become huge. Enlargement of the left atrium is detected most readily by a barium swallow

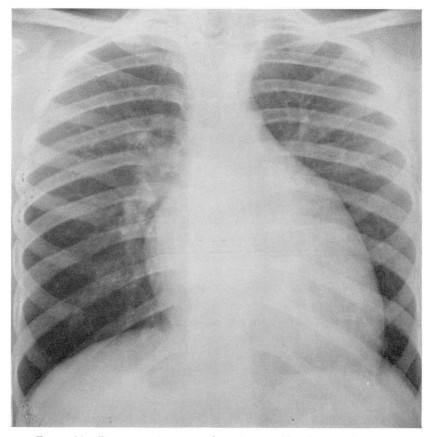

Figure 26. Posteroanterior view of a 10 year old girl with rheumatic heart disease and mitral insufficiency. There is marked left ventricular enlargement.

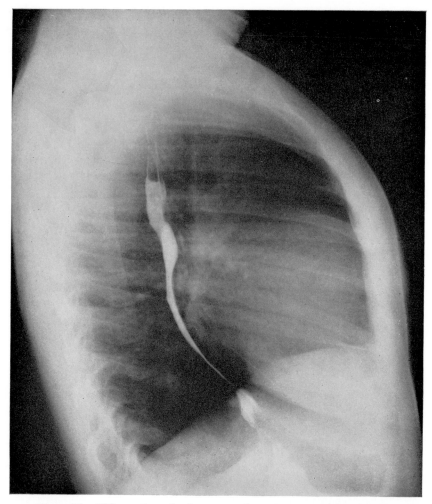

Figure 27.   Oblique view of a barium swallow of a 10 year old girl with mitral insufficiency. The enlarged left auricle has displaced the esophagus posteriorly.

with the patient in the erect position. In the right anterior oblique view, the enlarged left atrium displaces the esophagus posteriorly (Fig. 27). An enlarged left atrium sometimes causes a double density along the right cardiac border and, when marked, displaces the left main bronchus upward. Although the barium-filled esophageal view is the most reliable method, care must be taken to avoid a false positive interpretation: the barium should coat both walls of the esophagus, the degree of rotation should be optimal, and the film should be taken in inspiration. It is often necessary to monitor the procedure with fluoroscopy. Occasionally, marked enlargement of the left ventricle may displace the barium posteriorly and give the erroneous impression of left atrial enlargement.

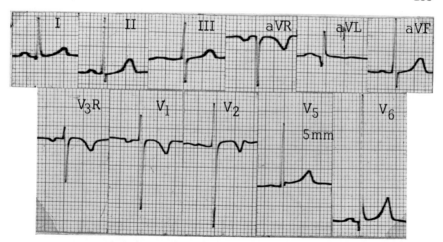

Figure 28. Electrocardiogram of a 10 year old girl with rheumatic heart disease and mitral insufficiency. Broad P waves denote left auricular hypertrophy. Deep S waves in leads V_1 and V_2 and tall R waves in leads V_5 and V_6 indicate left ventricular hypertrophy.

Electrocardiogram

The majority of children with mitral regurgitation have normal electrocardiograms. In patients with moderate or severe regurgitation, the electrocardiogram reflects enlargement of the left atrium and left ventricle (Fig. 28). The P wave is widened and has a flat top. It is not uncommonly inverted or diphasic in lead V_1 with a sharp, deep downstroke (Arevalo et al., 1963). In more advanced cases there may be ST and T wave changes over the left side of the precordium. Pulmonary hypertension is a late complication of mitral insufficiency and occurs rarely in childhood. However, when pulmonary hypertension is present, right ventricular hypertrophy may occur.

MITRAL STENOSIS

Pathology

Several pathologic mechanisms may be involved in the development of mitral stenosis. Brock (1952) has suggested that the most significant initial event is fusion of the valve cusps at the two opposing critical areas of tendon insertion. Adhesions between the cusps may occur even when the valvulitis is mild, causing a slight reduction in the size of the mitral aperture. This is usually of no functional importance. However, the mitral orifice may continue to decrease in size with time, possibly by the deposition of fibrin and platelets (Magarey, 1951). Thus severe stenosis may occur ultimately following an apparently mild attack of valvulitis.

In patients with more severe valvulitis, in addition to the valve cusps, the chordae tendineae, the atrioventricular ring, and even the papillary muscles are involved in the inflammatory process. The chordae tendineae become thickened and fused. The movement of the valves is restricted and increases the degree of stenosis. Since the valves cannot seal during systole, mitral regurgitation also occurs. Different grades of severity and the unequal involvement of various portions of the valve structure cause different end results. It is not surprising, therefore, that various degrees and combinations of mitral regurgitation and stenosis are found clinically.

Most observers in this country believe that functionally significant mitral stenosis does not usually occur in less than 2 to 3 years following an acute attack and more commonly 5 to 20 years elapse. Mitral stenosis is more common among children in other countries and stenosis appears to develop more rapidly. Reale and his associates (1963) reported a series of 54 symptomatic young patients with mitral stenosis from Italy. The patients ranged from 8 to 15 years of age and the interval of time between the first known attack of rheumatic fever and the onset of symptoms averaged 2 years with a minimum of 6 months.

Hemodynamic Effects

A diastolic pressure gradient across the mitral valve develops as the obstruction to blood flow at the mitral orifice increases. The pressure in the left atrium rises to overcome this gradient and this chamber hypertrophies. The increased left atrial pressure is transmitted back to the pulmonary capillary network which becomes engorged. As the pulmonary capillary pressure rises, arteriolar resistance increases and pulmonary hypertension develops. The pressure load on the right ventricle increases, leading to hypertrophy of this chamber. The work of the left ventricle is either normal or reduced unless there is concomitant mitral or aortic regurgitation.

Clinical Findings

Exertional dyspnea, hemoptysis, and attacks of acute pulmonary edema may occur if the stenosis is severe. The precordium is full and a right ventricular tap is palpable. The auscultatory signs of mitral stenosis are a loud first heart sound, an accentuated pulmonary component of the second sound, an opening snap, and an apical diastolic rumble at the apex. All of these findings are not always present simultaneously in children.

The loud ringing first heart sound may be the first sign of a developing stenosis. The first heart sound is loud because with mitral stenosis the valve cusps are depressed further into the ventricular cavity increasing the force and degree of movement toward the atrium as ventricular contraction occurs (Dack et al., 1960).

The opening snap is heard best in patients with pure mitral stenosis and is detected therefore less frequently in children. It is thought to be due to the sudden arrest of the downward movement of the thickened mitral leaflets (Dack et al., 1960). The opening snap occurs immediately after the second sound and has a high-pitched clicking quality. It is often heard best midway between the apex and the left sternal border.

The characteristic auscultatory finding of mitral stenosis is the low-pitched rumbling diastolic murmur accentuated in presystole by the increased pressure of atrial contraction. In patients with mitral regurgitation who are developing stenosis, the mid-diastolic murmur becomes longer, and as the obstruction increases, the presystolic component emerges. The diastolic rumble is often localized to a small area just inside the cardiac apex. It is heard best with the patient during the act of turning to the left lateral decubitus position with the bell portion of the stethoscope held lightly against the chest wall (Levine and Harvey, 1959). Exercise may accentuate the murmur and bring out its presystolic crescendo quality.

In children with mitral valvular disease the predominant lesion is usually mitral regurgitation and it is often difficult to decide clinically if mitral stenosis is also present. A pansystolic murmur occurs in combined mitral disease. A short mid-diastolic murmur is common in patients with pure regurgitation and it may be confused with the diastolic murmur heard in mitral stenosis. An opening snap may also be present with both lesions but it is much more frequent in mitral stenosis. On the other hand a third heart sound is associated with regurgitation and is virtually never heard when hemodynamically significant mitral stenosis exists. Radiographic and electrocardiographic examinations may be helpful in assessing the significance of a systolic murmur in patients with mitral stenosis, but not infrequently cardiac catheterization and angiocardiographic studies are necessary (Ross et al., 1958).

Radiologic Findings

Radiographic changes in mitral stenosis depend on the degree of stenosis. Since established mitral stenosis is rare in childhood, the findings are usually minimal, showing only a small heart with straightening of the upper left cardiac border (Fig. 29). Not infrequently, even if the stenosis is severe, the cardiac silhouette may not be enlarged. Slight left atrial enlargement is an early sign and is indicated by an indentation of the upper part of the barium-filled esophagus. The more characteristic x-ray findings associated with left atrial enlargement occur later (Fig. 30). In more advanced cases associated with pulmonary hypertension, right ventricular enlargement occurs, characterized in the posteroanterior view by eleva-

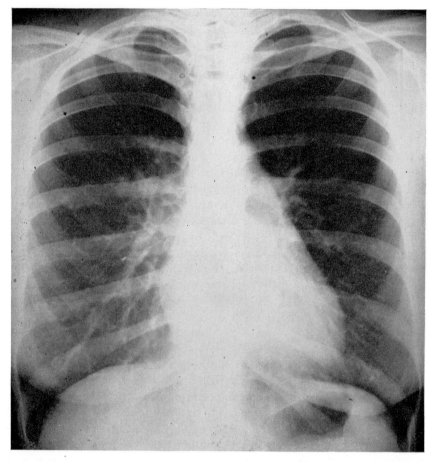

Figure 29. Posteroanterior view of a 15 year old girl with rheumatic heart disease and mitral stenosis. Heart is not enlarged but the left cardiac border is straightened.

tion of the cardiac apex above the diaphragm. Straightening or bulging of the cardiac waist due to a combination of dilatation of the pulmonary artery and hypertrophy of the right ventricular outflow tract also occurs (Fig. 31). The left ventricle is not enlarged unless there is associated aortic or mitral regurgitation.

Electrocardiogram

The tracing is usually normal in children with mild mitral stenosis. The earliest electrocardiographic abnormality is limited to the P waves which become broad and notched. In the more severe cases, right axis deviation and right ventricular hypertrophy develop (Fig. 32). Left ven-

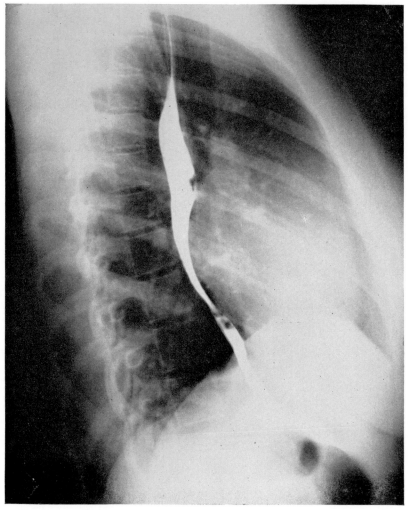

Figure 30. Oblique view of a barium swallow of a 14 year old girl with mitral stenosis. The enlarged left atrium has displaced the esophagus posteriorly.

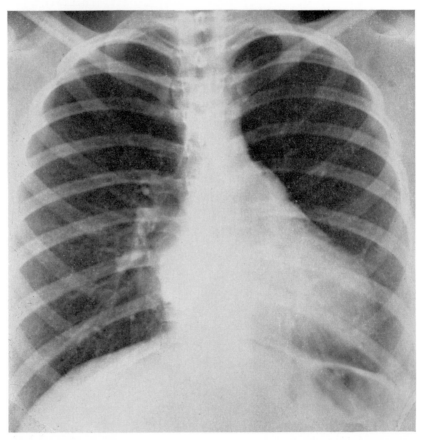

Figure 31.   Posteroanterior view of a 14 year old girl with rheumatic heart disease and mitral stenosis. There is right ventricular enlargement with upward and outward displacement of the apex and a prominence of the main pulmonary artery.

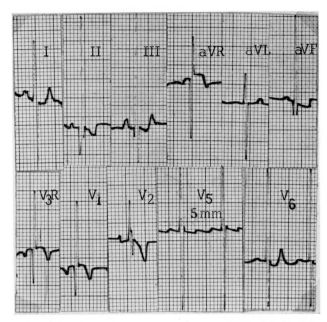

Figure 32. Electrocardiogram of a 14 year old girl with mitral stenosis. Notched P wave in lead I denotes left auricular hypertrophy. Deep Q waves and tall R waves in leads V₃R and V₁ indicate right ventricular hypertrophy.

tricular hypertrophy may occur if there is combined mitral stenosis and regurgitation.

AORTIC REGURGITATION

Pathology

Acute aortic valvulitis can cause mild regurgitation in the early phase of the disease which may then disappear as the inflammatory process heals. More often, signs of aortic regurgitation become apparent later in the course of the acute attack and usually persist thereafter. Severe inflammation of the valves leads to thickening and shortening of the cusps, and permanent incompetence results. A minor degree of fusion of the leaflets may occur but significant aortic stenosis takes years to develop and is very rare in childhood.

Hemodynamic Effects

Aortic incompetence allows blood to regurgitate back into the left ventricle during diastole. Most of the reflux occurs early in diastole and the stream of blood rushing back causes the characteristic diastolic murmur. The regurgitant flow in addition to the blood arriving from the left atrium increases the volume load in the left ventricle and this chamber dilates, often to huge proportions. The diastolic pressure is depressed and the systolic pressure increases to maintain a normal mean arterial pressure. To compensate for the regurgitating blood, a much larger stroke volume is required to maintain cardiac output. The abrupt ejection of the increased ventricular stroke volume causes a vigorous bounding pulse wave in the peripheral arteries. As the arterial pressure decreases rapidly with the regurgitation of blood, the pulse wave drops precipitously, causing the water-hammer type of pulse.

Clinical Findings

When aortic insufficiency first appears, the clinical signs are limited to a diastolic murmur. The blood pressure is normal and there are no peripheral signs. As the severity increases, the diagnosis can be suspected from the peripheral vascular signs. The systolic blood pressure rises and the diastolic pressure falls. Visible pulsations may be noted in the suprasternal notch and in the neck vessels. The radial pulse strikes the finger suddenly and falls away rapidly (Corrigan's pulse). When the pulse is auscultated over the femoral artery a booming "pistol shot" is heard during systole. If the bell of the stethoscope is pressed against the artery, a systolic and diastolic murmur may be heard (Duroziez's sign). Capillary pulsations may be visible in the nail beds and in the eyegrounds.

In children with moderate to severe aortic insufficiency the heart is enlarged. The apical impulse is displaced downward and to the left. Often a left ventricular heave is visible. The characteristic diastolic murmur of aortic regurgitation is grade 2/6 to 4/6 in intensity. It begins immediately after the second sound, has a high-pitched blowing quality, and has a decrescendo configuration. It is usually maximal in the second left intercostal space and is referred downward along the left sternal border. It may sometimes be heard at the apex. Occasionally, it is maximal in the second right intercostal space. It is best heard with the diaphragm of the stethoscope with the patient sitting or leaning forward with the breath held in expiration. An ejection systolic murmur is usually audible over the aortic area because of the rapid ejection of blood into the aorta. A systolic click may also be present and is caused by a large stroke volume entering the dilated aorta. A late diastolic murmur may be heard at the apex (Austin Flint murmur). This murmur is due to vibrations produced in the mitral valve by the aortic regurgitant stream (Ross and Criley, 1964). The Austin Flint murmur may be confused with the murmur of organic mitral stenosis (Segal et al., 1958). However, this is not a common diagnostic dilemma in pediatrics, since both the Austin Flint murmur and organic mitral stenosis are encountered much less frequently in children than in adults.

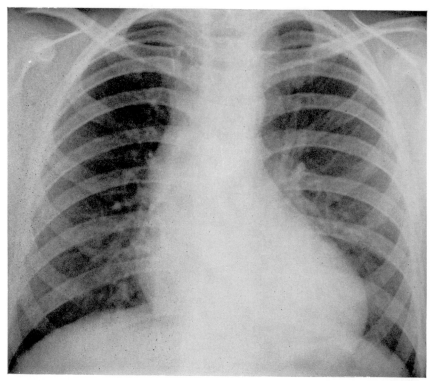

Figure 33. Posteroanterior view of a 12 year old boy with rheumatic heart disease and aortic insufficiency. Note left ventricular enlargement and widened aortic shadow.

Roentgenographic Findings

The x-ray findings are characterized by an enlarged left ventricle with an increase in the cardiothoracic index, elongation of the left ventricular contour, and downward displacement of the apex (Fig. 33). The ascending portion of the aorta is dilated and widens the shadow to the right of the sternum. The aortic knob may be prominent.

Electrocardiogram

The early changes associated with aortic insufficiency are increased voltage of the QRS complexes and deep Q waves over the left side of the precordium (Fig. 34). The T waves become tall and peaked in V_5 and V_6, the so-called diastolic overload pattern (Cabrera et al., 1952). More marked signs of left ventricular hypertrophy appear subsequently, and in the more advanced cases, a left ventricular strain pattern with depressed ST segments and inverted T waves may occur (Fig. 35).

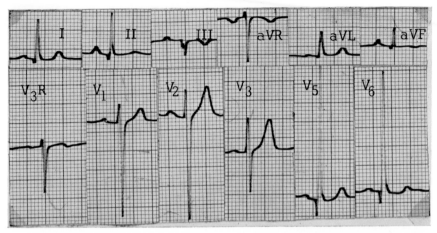

Figure 34. Electrocardiogram of a 13 year old boy with rheumatic heart disease and aortic insufficiency. Deep S waves in lead V_1 and tall R waves and prominent Q waves in leads V_5 and V_6 denote left ventricular hypertrophy.

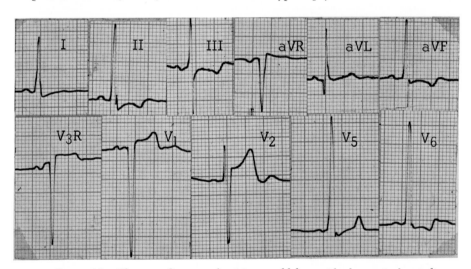

Figure 35. Electrocardiogram of a 14 year old boy with rheumatic heart disease and aortic insufficiency. There is evidence of left ventricular hypertrophy and strain.

MANAGEMENT

Medical Treatment

The medical management of children with chronic rheumatic heart disease involves: (1) the institution and maintenance of antistreptococcal prophylaxis to prevent recurrent attacks (page 128), (2) the treatment of congestive heart failure (page 110), (3) the regulation of physical activities (page 113), and (4) prophylactic measures to prevent subacute bacterial endocarditis (page 167). These subjects are discussed in other sections of the monograph.

Surgical Treatment

Great strides have been made in surgical techniques for the relief of rheumatic valvular disease. Experience with these techniques has been obtained mainly from the treatment of adults. Children are much less often severely disabled from rheumatic valvular disease. When they are, the heart is often very large, active rheumatic myocarditis is suspected, and they are not usually considered suitable candidates for surgery. Nevertheless, the occasional child or young adolescent is encountered in whom chronic valvular disease is the cause of severe congestive failure and in whom surgical intervention should be seriously considered. As methods improve, the indications for operation will undoubtedly be broadened to include young patients with valvular disease before severe enlargement and intractable failure occurs.

Mitral Regurgitation. Incompetence of the mitral valve is a common and fairly benign lesion in childhood. However, some children develop such severe regurgitation that the heart enlarges greatly and the patient is severely handicapped. Before open heart surgery was developed, no surgical procedure was available. Now, however, correction of this defect is possible.

Recently, Noonan and Spencer (1964) presented data on 3 adolescents with mitral insufficiency in whom valvular replacement was performed. Stern and his associates (1964) reported 4 patients, ages 6 to 16 years, in whom mitral annuloplasty resulted in marked improvement. Yuan et al. (1964) reported successful mitral annuloplasty in an 11 year old boy with severe regurgitation and atrial fibrillation. These authors suggested the following criteria as a basis for selection of patients with inactive rheumatic heart disease: (a) congestive heart failure not controlled by medical therapy, (b) progressive severe left atrial and left ventricular enlargement, and (c) pulmonary hypertension. The surgical procedure of choice depends on the anatomical derangements found at operation. It is not yet possible to judge results of valve replacement.

Mitral Stenosis. Severe mitral stenosis is rare in childhood in this country. It does, however, occur and commissurotomy has proved successful in children (Lurie and Shumacker, 1954; Brest et al., 1959; Gray, 1958; Castle and Baylin, 1961). Fairly large series of patients have been reported from other countries (Angelino et al., 1956; Borman et al., 1961; Gilbert-Queralto et al., 1962; Reale et al., 1963).

Surgery is indicated in young patients with mitral stenosis who have progressive dyspnea on exertion, attacks of pulmonary edema, paroxysmal dyspnea, or severe pulmonary hypertension. In selecting patients for surgery, a careful assessment must be made of the severity of the stenosis, the state of the myocardium, and the presence and degree of mitral regurgitation. It is often necessary to perform hemodynamic and angiocardiographic studies to evaluate the degree of regurgitation and stenosis (Marshall et al., 1958; Bjork et al., 1960).

A detailed discussion of the various surgical procedures and the indications for open versus closed valvulotomy is beyond the scope of this monograph (Kay and Zimmerman, 1962). Open valvulotomy is being employed more frequently and this may become the procedure of choice in children since it is often necessary to deal with an associated mitral regurgitation.

The reported results of mitral valvulotomy in children have in general been good. Recurrent stenosis in adults is common (Ellis, 1964). However, the incidence of re-stenosis in children is not yet known. There is no evidence that intervening rheumatic recurrences are related to the occurrence of re-stenosis.

Aortic Regurgitation. The surgical treatment of aortic regurgitation is still in the experimental stage. Valvular prostheses are currently being used and good short-term results have been reported. Valvular replacement has been performed rarely in children and it is too early to assess results (Noonan and Spencer, 1964).

COMPLICATIONS

SUBACUTE BACTERIAL ENDOCARDITIS

Subacute bacterial endocarditis is a very serious, potentially lethal complication of rheumatic heart disease. Before the advent of antibiotics the mortality rate was nearly 100 per cent. At the present time with the use of penicllin, streptomycin, and Staphcillin, the mortality rate has been reduced to 30 to 40 per cent (Kerr, 1964).

Incidence

Subacute bacterial endocarditis is less common in rheumatic children than in rheumatic adults. Bacterial endocarditis usually does not develop until several years after the initial rheumatic episode. Since the peak incidence of the first rheumatic attack is at the age of 8 years, bacterial endocarditis is uncommon in rheumatic children less than 10 years old.

During the past 40 years the incidence of subacute bacterial endocarditis in rheumatic children has remained essentially the same. In 1928 Schlesinger in a series of 349 autopsies of rheumatic children reported 10 cases of subacute bacterial endocarditis, an incidence of 2.8 per cent. In 1942, Jones and Bland reported 15 cases of subacute bacterial endocarditis in 653 rheumatic children (2.3 per cent) followed for 10 years. In 1948 Ash in a similar study observed 12 cases among 318 rheumatic children (3.7 per cent) also during a 10 year period.

In a 13 year period, 1944 to 1956, Cutler et al. (1958) reported 8 cases of subacute bacterial endocarditis in rheumatic children and 1 case in a boy with combined rheumatic and congenital heart disease. During a 28 year period, 1931 to 1959, Blumenthal et al. (1960) reported 17 cases of subacute bacterial endocarditis in rheumatic children and 1 case in a boy with combined rheumatic and congenital heart disease. In 1 of these patients the infection followed a dental extraction, and in another dental caries was noted. In the remaining 16 patients no data on a possible portal of entry could be obtained.

Portal of Entry

In the majority of cases of subacute bacterial endocarditis the portal of entry cannot be identified. However, it has been well documented that transient bacteremia occurs frequently after dental extractions and tonsillectomies. Robinson et al. (1950) reported studies on blood cultures taken on 599 patients after dental extractions. Blood cultures obtained immediately after the procedure were positive in 39 per cent. If several teeth were removed at one time, the number of positive cultures rose to 73 per cent. In the opinion of this observer, the incidence of positive cultures was not increased by the presence of dental infection or the amount of operative trauma. Taran (1944) reported an incidence of 52 per cent after dental extractions in 350 rheumatic children. Four of these patients (1.1 per cent) developed subacute bacterial endocarditis. Elliott (1939), in a series of 100 patients, reported 38 positive blood cultures following tonsillectomy.

Bacteriology

The great majority of cases are due to alpha streptococci. Gamma streptococci and enterococci (Lancefield group D) and staphylococci occur less frequently. Occasionally gram-negative bacilli such as *H. influenzae* and members of the enteric group cause these infections.

Prevention

Transient bacteremia occurs frequently after dental extractions or tonsillectomy. It has also been observed after instrumentation of the genitourinary tract, surgery of the intestinal tract, and childbirth. Therefore before such procedures are undertaken or at the time of parturition, every rheumatic individual should receive antibiotic prophylaxis to prevent implantation of these organisms in diseased cardiac valves.

Sulfonamide drugs are of no value for this purpose. Penicillin is the drug of choice. Rheumatic individuals taking daily oral prophylactic penicillin represent a special problem because this medication may have eliminated penicillin-sensitive organisms, and the remaining strains are frequently penicillin-resistant (Garrod and Waterworth, 1962). Hook and Kaye (1962) have suggested that it might be advisable to omit the usual daily doses of prophylactic penicillin for a few days. Broad-spectrum antibiotics are less effective than penicillin because they may not penetrate the fibrin nidus surrounding the bacterial implant, and the organisms therefore are not eradicated.

Treatment Schedules for Prevention of Subacute Bacterial Endocarditis: Regimens Recommended by the American Heart Association.

DAY OF PROCEDURE. Procaine penicillin 600,000 units supplemented by 600,000 units crystalline penicillin 1 to 2 hours before the procedure.

Intramuscular penicillin is more reliable. However, because of practical considerations, some dentists and physicians rely on oral penicillin when the full cooperation of the patient is assured. If oral penicillin is to be employed on the day of procedure, 4 doses (every 4 to 6 hours) of at least 0.25 gram of alpha-phenoxymethyl penicillin (Penicillin V) or alpha-phenoxyethyl penicillin (phenethicillin), or 500,000 units of buffered penicillin G should be given; in addition, an extra dose should be taken 1 hour before the procedure.

FOR TWO DAYS AFTER PROCEDURE. Procaine penicillin 600,000 units intramuscularly each day. In selected instances, 0.25 gram of alpha-phenoxymethyl penicillin (Penicillin V), or alpha-phenoxyethyl penicillin (phenethicillin), or 500,000 units of buffered penicillin G 4 times daily by mouth on each day may be used for those patients in whom full cooperation is anticipated and ingestion is assured.

CONTRAINDICATIONS TO THIS REGIMEN. The main contraindication is sensitivity to penicillin. All patients should be carefully questioned for previous history suggesting penicillin sensitivity. If such a history is obtained, even if equivocal, penicillin should not be given. Under such circumstances, erythromycin should be used in a dose of 250 mg. by mouth 4 times daily for adults and older children. For small children, a dose of 20 mg. per pound per day divided into 3 or 4 evenly spaced doses may be used. The total dose should not exceed 1 gram per day.

Instrumentation of Genitourinary Tract, Surgery of the Lower Intestinal Tract, and Childbirth. With these procedures, transitory bacteremia due to penicillin-resistant enterococci is apt to occur. The use of penicillin alone in the doses suggested cannot be expected to curtail bacteremia due to enterococci, a common cause of bacterial endocarditis.

For these reasons, it is suggested that, as an empirical guide, the aforementioned intramuscular penicillin regimen be used in combination with streptomycin 1 or 2 grams intramuscularly on the day of the procedure and for each of two days following the procedure. In children, streptomycin may be given in a dosage of 50 mg./kg., not to exceed 1 gram per day. In patients who are sensitive to penicillin, a combination of erythromycin and streptomycin or a broad-spectrum antibiotic combined with streptomycin may be of some use, although it should be emphasized that very little information is available about these antibiotic combinations and their efficacy in preventing bacterial endocarditis due to enterococci.

Diagnosis of Subacute Bacterial Endocarditis in Rheumatic Individuals

Subacute bacterial endocarditis should be suspected in every rheumatic individual with unexplained low-grade fever. Even if other characteristic signs of subacute bacterial endocarditis are lacking, blood cultures should be taken because prompt treatment is extremely important and failure to recognize this complication is all too common. The differentiation of a rheumatic recurrence from subacute bacterial endocarditis is often difficult. Characteristic signs of the latter are petechiae, clubbing, and splenomegaly. Arthralgias and red blood cells occur in both diseases. Osler's nodes occur occasionally in subacute bacterial endocarditis and are diagnostic (Blumenthal et al., 1960). Splinter hemorrhages and Janeway's lesions occur too infrequently in children to be of aid in the differential diagnosis. Erythema marginatum and subcutaneous nodules do not occur in subacute bacterial endocarditis and are characteristic of rheumatic fever. An elevated ASO titer also suggests that the symptoms may be due to a rheumatic recurrence.

The diagnosis of subacute bacterial endocarditis is confirmed by blood culture. As soon as the diagnosis is suspected, repeated blood cultures should be taken and therapy begun after 24 to 36 hours without waiting for the laboratory results. In taking the blood cultures, the amount of blood added to the culture medium is important (Robinson et al., 1950). Five ml. of blood added to 100 ml. of broth is more likely to give positive results than larger amounts of blood added to the same volume of medium. However, despite the most careful technique, blood cultures obtained from some patients with typical clinical findings remain sterile. In such cases, although the causative organism remains unidentified, vigorous therapy with several different antibiotic agents should be started.

Therapy

Penicillin is undoubtedly the drug of choice in practically all cases of subacute bacterial endocarditis because of its clot-penetrating, bactericidal properties and low toxicity (Tumulty, 1962). Peaks of penicillin are preferable to the maintenance of a sustained level because bacteria are most susceptible during the logarithmic phase of growth. According to Tumulty 1 million units of penicillin per day given in divided doses will give a blood level of about 1 unit. Five to 10 times the amount of penicillin needed to inhibit the growth of the organism, as determined by sensitivity tests, should be given daily. Oral penicillin is not recommended because of variations in absorption. The addition of streptomycin to penicillin is thought to increase the bactericidal properties of penicillin. With highly sensitive organisms 4 weeks of treatment is usually sufficient. With infections due to pneumococci or enterococci which have a destructive action on the valvular tissue, therapy should be continued for 6 to 8 weeks. If the infection is due to *Staphylococcus aureus*, Staphcillin should be given.

ATRIAL FIBRILLATION

Atrial fibrillation rarely occurs during an acute attack of rheumatic carditis. In patients with chronic rheumatic heart disease this complication is less common in children than in adults (Gibson, 1941). The prognosis of patients who develop this complication is always poor. Among 441 children and adolescents Feinstein et al. (1964) observed atrial fibrillation in 9 patients (2 per cent). Six of these 9 patients died during an 8 year period.

PULMONARY COMPLICATIONS

A bacterial or viral pneumonia not infrequently precipitates congestive heart failure in patients with chronic rheumatic heart disease, and it is also a common complication of patients already in failure. Patients with mitral stenosis are especially susceptible to lower respiratory infections. Pneumonia was one of the major causes of death among young adults during the 1957-1958 outbreak of Asian influenza. Giles and Shuttleworth (1957) reported 7 patients with rheumatic valvular disease among 46 deaths associated with influenza. In a study of fatal cases in the Netherlands, there were 10 individuals with mitral stenosis (Hers and Mulder, 1961). The effects of infections due to influenza viruses on the cardiovascular system have been reviewed by Medearis and his associates (1963).

Vaccines for a number of viral agents are now available. Because of the increased risk of serious complications, vaccination is recommended for patients with severe chronic rheumatic heart disease, especially during epidemics.

Chapter Fifteen

COMMUNITY HEALTH SERVICES

By Leon Gordis, M.D.

INTRODUCTION

Mortality from both acute rheumatic fever and rheumatic heart disease has declined steadily over the years, but these conditions nevertheless continue to constitute serious public health problems in the United States and in many parts of the world. In 1960, for example, 18,411 deaths in the United States were due to rheumatic fever and chronic rheumatic heart disease. These conditions accounted for 1.1 per cent of all deaths in this country, with a death rate of 10.3 per 100,000 population (U.S. Dept. H.E.W., Public Health Service, 1964). In 1954, the Framingham study of heart disease in adults (Stokes and Dawber, 1956) found a prevalence rate for rheumatic heart disease of 24 per 1000 adults ages 30 to 39. A recent study of rheumatic fever and rheumatic heart disease among entering U.S. college students (Marienfeld et al., 1964) revealed a national prevalence rate for rheumatic fever of 17.5 per 1000 college students examined, and ranged from 6.3 to 39.5 per 1000 when analyzed according to individual states of residence. The national rate for rheumatic heart disease was 5.7 per 1000 and ranged from 2.0 to 12.3 in the individual states. From the data obtained in this study, the Heart Disease Control Program of the U.S. Public Health Service estimates conservatively that at least 665,000 people in the United States suffer from rheumatic fever or rheumatic heart disease.

The full impact of rheumatic fever and its sequelae must be measured not by statistics alone, but also in terms of the toll it may take throughout the life of each victim of the disease. Physical limitation, eventual incapacitation, and early death are often the lot of the patient with rheumatic heart disease. Restricted employment opportunities and decreased insurability are but two of the many associated problems which result from the actual physical handicap. The disability resulting from rheumatic fever, however, is much more extensive than that resulting from organic heart disease alone. Since rheumatic fever is most common in school-age children, the emotional problems generated by prolonged hospitalization and convalescence and the associated social and educational deprivation are particularly critical. The long-term emotional and social difficulties resulting from chronic disease in childhood have not been adequately studied but are no doubt considerable. These aspects of rheumatic fever, although not easily tabulated or analyzed statistically, are painfully real to the physician who is responsible for the care of rheumatic children and follows their course during childhood, adolescence, and beyond.

In purely financial terms the cost to the community of rheumatic fever and rheumatic heart disease is staggering. A survey conducted by the Minnesota Department of Health (Mathy, 1958) showed that in 1957 $175,000 was spent in the state for medical expenses and hospitalization resulting only from *recurrences* of acute rheumatic fever. This study estimated that 90 per cent of these recurrences could have been prevented by a statewide secondary prophylaxis program costing $20,000 a year. As of September 1961, 38,786 veterans were receiving compensation for rheumatic fever and rheumatic heart disease with a total value of over 2.3 million dollars a year.

Thus rheumatic fever and rheumatic heart disease constitute major public health problems today because of their great impact on the afflicted individual and his community. Furthermore, successful control and prevention of these diseases require a multi-faceted approach by many medical and paramedical personnel in addition to the practicing physician. The skills of state and local health officers, public health nurses, social workers, health educators, and laboratory technicians are all necessary. Identifying rheumatic patients and maintaining them on long-term prophylaxis against streptococcal infections depend on a cooperative community-wide program of action by official, voluntary, and private agencies as well as by medical institutions and physicians in practice. In this chapter some major elements of such a community program will be reviewed.*

* A guide for public health personnel, *Services for Children with Heart Disease and Rheumatic Fever*, is available from the American Public Health Association, Inc., 1790 Broadway, New York 19, New York.

PRIMARY PREVENTION

Primary prevention is defined as the prevention of initial attacks of rheumatic fever. The association of antecedent group A streptococcal pharyngitis with this disease is universally accepted. Studies have shown that adequate treatment of these infections can reduce the incidence of rheumatic fever. Primary prevention today is therefore entirely confined to prompt detection and adequate treatment of all such infections (Chapter 13). No other means is presently known to prevent initial attacks of rheumatic fever.

Case Finding

Prevention of initial attacks of rheumatic fever in a community depends on a well organized continuous program of case finding—a term denoting both detection of patients with streptococcal infections and adequate follow-up. Although many children with respiratory illness are brought to the private physician or clinic promptly, they do not always have the benefit of the modern diagnostic methods available for identifying beta hemolytic streptococci. Many others whose general medical care is episodic often do not receive immediate attention. Since rheumatic fever is primarily a disease of school-age children and has a high incidence in lower socio-economic groups whose medical care is often inadequate, the parents, school nurse, and public health nurse have a vital role in the early identification of such children with respiratory infections and in referring them for proper diagnosis and medical treatment.

Case identification is of little value, however, without proper follow-through for diagnosis and treatment. The nurse should not be satisfied with having referred the child for care, but must subsequently see that medical attention has been sought *and* obtained, find out what therapy if any has been prescribed, and see that it is taken for the necessary period. Many cases of rheumatic fever result from failure of patients to take the full 10 day course of oral penicillin prescribed by their physicians, particularly in busy clinics where the doctor-patient relationship is unfortunately hurried and impersonal (Bergman and Werner, 1963). This problem offers an ideal opportunity for the public health nurse to provide the essential link for successful disease prevention. Even when home care is good, therapy is often discontinued as soon as the clinical symptoms subside, despite explicit instructions by the physician to take penicillin for a full 10 days.

Diagnostic Facilities

Proper diagnostic services must be available in each community. In addition to medical examinations by private or clinic physicians, facilities for throat cultures should be available. Bacteriologic laboratory facilities may be in private laboratories, in a health department or hospital, or as has been shown feasible, in the practicing physician's own office (Markowitz, 1963). It is not difficult for a physician to learn how to identify properly colonies of β hemolytic streptococci on blood agar plates. For physicians who prefer to use health department facilities, packets containing Dacron-tipped swabs can be mailed conveniently. Various communities have established fluorescent antibody (FA) laboratories for the detection of group A streptococci (Warfield et al., 1961; Moody et al., 1963). The FA method is rapid and a telephone report can usually be made to the physician within a few hours after the swab arrives at the laboratory. The method is expensive, however, requiring a trained technician and special reagents and equipment, so that the advisability of establishing an FA laboratory for streptococcal identification must be decided individually for each community. Once an FA laboratory is established in a community, however, the technique can be easily applied to the identification of many other organisms, such as enteropathogenic *E. coli* and *C. diphtheriae*.

Education

Physician education is important in community primary prevention programs. Since in many instances the diagnosis of a streptococcal pharyngitis cannot be made clinically, the use of throat cultures must be stressed. In some areas physicians are not yet fully aware of the importance of 10 full days of penicillin therapy for eradication of streptococci. The physician must realize that the same regimen of antibiotic therapy may not be suitable for different families. Some families may never have a prescription filled because of the expense. Others cannot be depended upon to continue 10 days of oral therapy under any circumstances, and intramuscular administration may be indicated. In busy clinics, in particular, the background information on the family gathered by the public health nurse and social worker is often invaluable in deciding on the form of therapy to be instituted and indeed may in some cases be decisive for the success of treatment and the consequent prevention of rheumatic fever.

A broad program of public education is also necessary to alert parents to consult physicians when their children have sore throats. Such programs are often effectively conducted through schools, parent-teacher associations, and other community groups, as well as through mass media.

SECONDARY PREVENTION

Secondary prevention denotes prevention of rheumatic recurrences in individuals who have had an attack of rheumatic fever, and depends on a program of continuous antimicrobial prophylaxis in rheumatic patients. Repeated attacks of rheumatic fever are the chief cause of progressive cardiac damage in rheumatic fever patients. The decline in the number of patients with severe rheumatic heart disease observed over the past 20 years reflects in large measure the introduction of secondary prevention programs in many communities. The accomplishments of these programs result from the combined efforts of physician, school nurse, public health nurse, social worker, and other personnel. Operation of these programs will be reviewed in this section.

Case Finding

All new cases of rheumatic fever must be identified so that proper preventive measures can be instituted promptly. Case finding of acute rheumatic fever is therefore an important responsibility of private and school physicians as well as public health nurses. Although overt cases of rheumatic fever are usually easily recognized, the onset in many patients is insidious. Loss of appetite, fatiguability, pallor, and weakness may be present for some time, and receive attention only when school performance deteriorates. The teacher or school nurse may be the first to suspect a medical basis for changes in a child's behavior or academic achievement. Intensified programs of health education should therefore be directed to teachers and school administrators who can prove instrumental in furthering case finding of rheumatic fever and many other health problems.

The need for case finding of rheumatic heart disease has led to the introduction of various methods for screening populations for heart disease. Morton et al. (1959) compared three such methods for detecting pediatric heart disease: a single lead (V_3R) electrocardiogram, a 70 mm. chest x-ray, and limited physical examination. Of the three methods used singly, greatest sensitivity and specificity were found with the physical examination. Equipment has recently been developed for screening children for heart disease through tape recordings of their heart sounds (Miller et al., 1962). Work is currently in progress to improve the efficiency of the system by using a computer for analysis of the recordings (Caceres et al., 1962). An important question yet to be answered is whether such screening projects for heart disease in children should be generally recommended for most communities.

Diagnostic Facilities

A referral system must be available for children suspected of having rheumatic fever and each community should provide or have easy access to good cardiac diagnostic facilities. This need can be partially met by practicing physicians, but cardiac diagnostic clinics are also needed. Such clinics can be established by the health department, local Heart Association, or other voluntary community agencies.

Since at present there is no single test diagnostic of rheumatic fever, diagnosis must be made on the basis of the modified Jones criteria. The number of cases of rheumatic fever which remain undiagnosed can be reduced by educating physicians in the use of these criteria. An even greater stimulus to such an educational program is the danger of over-diagnosis of rheumatic fever. Blackman (1963) studied 100 patients referred for consultation with a history of rheumatic fever and rheumatic heart disease, and found that in 35 the history of signs and symptoms did not satisfy the Jones criteria. He concluded that the referring physicians were not making adequate use of these criteria in their diagnoses. However, even among physicians who are aware of the importance of the Jones criteria as a diagnostic guide, misdiagnoses are made by incorrectly applying these criteria to individual cases. Grossman and Athreya (1962) studied 455 patients erroneously diagnosed as having rheumatic fever. The most common sources of error were misinterpretations of arthralgia as arthritis and of innocent or other nonrheumatic murmurs as rheumatic. In addition, physicians often considered an isolated minor criterion, such as fever, rise in antistreptolysin O titer, or elevated erythrocyte sedimentation rate, diagnostic of rheumatic fever.

Physician education must therefore emphasize both the importance of using the Jones criteria as a diagnostic guide and the proper way of applying them in clinical practice. Although rheumatic fever constitutes a significant community problem, the average practicing physician may see only one or two cases a year in his own practice. For this reason, any educational program concerned with diagnosis of rheumatic fever and directed to physicians must be continuous. A course given once, and lacking immediate clinical application, is rapidly forgotten.

A further measure to reduce the number of patients erroneously being treated as rheumatic is the periodic re-evaluation of rheumatic patients to identify those whose original diagnosis did not meet the Jones criteria and who should therefore be removed from prophylaxis. This procedure has been referred to as "delabeling" of rheumatic patients, and is especially important in view of the severe effects which result from the diagnosis of rheumatic fever even in the absence of any actual rheumatic disease. It is, of course, difficult for physicians to question the diagnosis of a patient who was cared for elsewhere during his acute episode. However, diagnostic re-evaluation is the physician's inescapable responsibility if many children and young people are to be spared unnecessary physical, social, and vocational restriction. In some cases it will be clear that the Jones criteria were never met, and attempts will have to be made to rescind the diagnosis. This may be difficult when a child has been considered and treated as rheumatic for some time, for his parents may find it hard to reorient their thinking and attitudes and change their handling of their child. They can be immeasurably assisted in this transition by the interest and guidance of an understanding public health nurse or medical social worker.

Physicians must accept the fact that many clinical conditions cannot be definitively diagnosed and may remain equivocal despite intensive diagnostic efforts. Overdiagnosis of rheumatic fever can be reduced by encouraging physicians to diagnose patients as "rheumatic suspects" when the diagnosis remains questionable even after properly applying the Jones criteria. Such a tentative diagnosis warrants prompt institution of prophylaxis, but also provides for thorough re-evaluation of the diagnosis after a specific interval.

Prophylactic Methods

After the acute attack has been treated, successful prevention depends entirely on continuous antimicrobial prophylaxis of streptococcal infections. Selection of an agent has been discussed in an earlier chapter (Chapter 12). Once an appropriate drug has been chosen it must be administered regularly as prescribed. The dose must be increased in the event of a breakthrough of infection, or when surgery or dental procedures, such as tooth extraction, are contemplated. Approximately 11 per cent of all cases of subacute bacterial endocarditis in patients with previous heart disease follow shortly after dental extraction (Robinson et al., 1950). Harvey et al. (1961) reported 5 cases of subacute bacterial endocarditis in rheumatic fever patients following various dental manipulations other than extraction. Educational programs for dentists must therefore stress the need for taking a proper history to uncover any previous rheumatic fever attack, and for antibiotic administration prior to and after the procedure. Education of physicians and dentists must also continually emphasize that although both sulfonamides and penicillin are effective in *preventing* streptococcal infection, sulfonamides are not effective in *treating* streptococcal infections, and treatment must be with penicillin or another antibiotic.

Comparative studies indicate that continuous prophylaxis with intramuscular penicillin is associated with a lower rate of rheumatic fever recurrences than is prophylaxis with oral preparations (Wood et al., 1964). This superiority may result entirely from the certainty of administration assured by monthly injections of penicillin. Some clinics use intramuscular penicillin prophylaxis exclusively in their secondary prevention programs.

The disadvantages of intramuscular penicillin include pain at the injection site and a slightly higher frequency of drug sensitization than with oral medication. Furthermore, some patients who drop out completely from an intramuscular penicillin program might have benefited from at least intermittent prophylaxis by irregular visits to a clinic offering oral penicillin. The choice of route should therefore be individualized for each patient, weighing many factors including age, interval since the last attack, and presence and severity of heart disease. Rheumatic fever recurrences are most frequent in patients who have residual heart disease (Taranta et al., 1964), and in these and other specific groups, intramuscular penicillin may be indicated. In addition, the social and family background may determine the regularity of drug administration in an oral program. As with primary prevention, the information obtained by the public health nurse and social worker may be important determinants of the regimen of prophylaxis finally selected by the physician.

Since rheumatic fever is most common among lower socio-economic groups living in crowded urban areas, preventive programs for this segment of the population can be effective only if medical facilities are available for long-term outpatient care in these areas. In addition to diagnostic centers, clinics must be established where those with marginal incomes can receive medical care and long-term prophylaxis. In contrast to many other outpatient services generally provided, clinics for rheumatic fever patients require special organization and staffing because of the close follow-up and long-term care involved. Such clinics must have public health nurses and social workers in addition to an augmented clerical staff. They must operate under enthusiastic and understanding physicians who are aware of the special problems involved in administering a secondary prevention program.

Drug Supply

Successful prophylaxis programs require ready availability of penicillin at modest cost. Many communities in the United States have prophylaxis programs sponsored by state or city health departments or by local Heart Association chapters. Many of these programs were established when the cost of long-term penicillin prophylaxis was prohibitive for most patients. Although the cost of penicillin has been considerably reduced since that time, there remains a need to ensure a continuous supply for rheumatic fever patients at reasonable cost, and at no cost for those unable to pay. In some areas the health department or Heart Association purchases penicillin in bulk and later resells it at cost to eligible patients. In other areas, pharmacists have agreed to sell penicillin at low cost to patients certified rheumatic by the responsible agency. The specific arrangement finally chosen must be individualized for each community. For such a program to succeed it must be a cooperative venture of all community organizations concerned. Although ultimately most of these programs become the administrative responsibility of a single agency, all those interested must share in the vital initial phases of program planning.

Case Registries

Agencies supplying penicillin inevitably become involved in some form of record keeping. In many states such records have evolved into case registries (U.S. Dept. H.E.W., Public Health Service, 1961; Saslaw et al., 1962; Branscome et al., 1963). A case registry represents an inventory of patients with a certain type of chronic problem to facilitate their care and supervision. The basic objective of a registry for rheumatic fever is to identify promptly those who are delinquent in their prophylaxis and medical supervision, so that they may be quickly restored to the program through an effective follow-up system. Other benefits may also accrue from a rheumatic fever registry, but they must always be considered secondary to this prime objective. Although most registries cannot serve as sources of reliable incidence and prevalence data, they may provide a gross estimate of the magnitude of the rheumatic fever problem in a community. In addition, the very existence of an active rheumatic fever registry in a community often increases public and professional aware-ness of the significance of the rheumatic fever problem, and focuses interest and attention on methods of control.

For a registry to function, however, it must generate physician interest and cooperation. To stimulate this response the registry and the sponsoring agency must render physicians some services in return. Such services may include supplying low-cost penicillin, distributing periodic reviews and analyses of the data accumulated by the registry, and establishing cardiac diagnostic facilities for those physicians who desire consultation. Experience has demonstrated that a registry must include a mechanism for the verification of diagnosis if its data are to be of value. The initial form on which the physician submits his patient's name to the registry should indicate which of the Jones criteria the case fulfilled. As these forms are received in the registry office, they should be reviewed by a physician, and if necessary, further clarification of the diagnosis should be secured through telephone call or letter. The verification procedure itself has proven to be a valuable measure for physician education in many communities. Although the prime objective of any registry is to maintain rheumatic fever patients on a program of continuous prophylaxis, in each instance the mechanics of the registry must be individualized to fit the needs of the community. A mechanism of program evaluation should be included, and its results continuously applied to improvement of the program and its services.

Failures in Secondary Prevention

Many recurrent attacks of rheumatic fever in the United States are in drop-outs from established prophylaxis programs. Considerable attention has therefore centered on the reasons for failure of continued prophylaxis and on possible remedies. As with many preventive medical programs, communicating the importance of secondary prophylaxis is difficult. At times, physicians themselves fail to appreciate the importance of continued long-term prophylaxis in an apparently well patient. Furthermore, it is difficult to convince a person who has recovered unscathed from his acute attack (and to convince his family as well) that although he is free of symptoms, he remains in a high-risk group in regard to recurrent attacks and future cardiac damage.

In order to reduce the number of drop-outs from secondary prevention programs, more time and personal attention must be given each patient by the physician and other clinic personnel. A patient's attitude toward his illness and his conception of the disease are closely related to his interest in and adherence to the prophylaxis program (Heinzelmann, 1962). The conception of the disease formed by the family of the rheumatic patient has been reported generally inadequate in families with gross conflicts, major recent social readjustments, or significant socio-economic deprivation (Elling et al., 1960). If the physician's attitude toward the mother indicated confidence in her reliability, strict adherence to the prophylactic regimen was more likely. Ambuel et al. (1964) found that in a general pediatric clinic broken appointments often related to how well the physician had conveyed the importance of the return visit. Thus, these studies indicate that the physician and other members of the clinic staff have a significant role in the regularity of follow-up of these patients. Awareness of the importance of his attitude and manner may enable the physician to modify his behavior so as to encourage greater patient cooperation.

The adolescent rheumatic continues to pose a major problem in discontinuance of prophylaxis. Adolescence is a period when numerous and varied changes occur very rapidly. The physical changes which follow puberty occur at the time the adolescent is developing new social and heterosexual relationships. Striving for independence from authority, he also has a great need for conformity with his peers. It is therefore not surprising that as the adolescent rheumatic struggles through this turbulent period, prophylactic medication is often discontinued. This may occur because of indifference or as part of his rejection of parental and medical authority as he attempts to establish independence of thought and action. In addition, the prospect of chronic physical illness confronts the adolescent with a painful situation which he cannot alter, but which he can and does try to avoid and forget.

Successful medical care of the adolescent therefore requires attitudes and approaches specifically designed for patients in this age group. The rheumatic adolescent must have the opportunity to discuss rheumatic fever and rheumatic heart disease with physicians and nurses from new points of view which begin to concern him, such as marriage and vocation. In addition to recognizing the unique problems and aspirations of the adolescent, the staff must make practical changes designed to maintain supervision at this precarious time. Adolescents should have the benefit of late afternoon or evening clinics. In addition, prophylaxis has a far better chance of success in this age group if the rheumatic problem is handled with other adolescent problems by a general adolescent clinic, rather than by a cardiac specialty or a pediatric clinic. Finally, special attention must be given to the serious discontinuity in medical care which confronts an adolescent in the transfer from pediatric to adult clinic. Many rheumatics never complete this transfer and are lost to medical care until their next rheumatic attack. Only by increased awareness and understanding of the adolescent and his problems, coupled with constructive action to facilitate his medical care, will greater success be achieved in maintaining this high-risk group on continuous prophylaxis.

ROLE OF THE PUBLIC HEALTH NURSE

Every phase of rheumatic fever control requires the participation of a public health nurse for maximal effectiveness. Through the services she provides, she becomes the main health consultant for many families who, recognizing her devotion and concern for them, have confidence in her and in her actions. This entree into the home is often an asset unique to the public health nurse, and it enables her to occupy an indispensable position in successful disease prevention and control programs. Prevention of rheumatic fever, for example, requires early case finding of streptococcal infection and is most effectively performed by the district public health nurse who serves a segment of the population which usually does not receive adequate medical care.

When hospitalization is indicated for a child during the acute attack, the public health nurse who has known the family members well can help allay their fears by a thorough discussion of the implications of the illness and the hospitalization. She may also be able to assist the family with the financial and personal problems which frequently accompany hospitalization. If convalescent care is subsequently needed, the public health nurse can be of great help in easing the transition to the convalescent unit and home. It has been pointed out (Dick and Grant, 1964) that of all the personnel involved in the care of the rheumatic patient, the public health nurse is the most frequently involved throughout the entire course of the disease, from the earliest suspicion of rheumatic fever and its subsequent diagnosis through convalescence and return to school or work. Thus, she can provide a major element of continuity so often missing in the care of patients with any chronic illness.

Much of the difficulty in maintaining prophylaxis stems from the patient's lack of clear understanding of the nature of rheumatic fever and why prophylaxis is needed. The public health nurse acts as health educator, supplying necessary knowledge and motivation for the patient to continue prophylaxis. Her home visits and close follow-up are another crucial factor in successful maintenance of prophylaxis. Through her evaluation of the home the prophylactic regimen as well as the entire medical approach can be individualized to the needs of the patient and his family. In some instances the nurse may arrange transportation to the clinic for a patient who would otherwise not attend. She may observe features of the home situation detrimental to the patient's health and remedy them. At other times, the home situation may be so fundamentally poor that only drastic changes in housing, employment, and other conditions may succeed in improving the patient's physical and emotional environment.

The public health nurse may also be instrumental in securing services such as home teaching when indicated. She may be an important liaison with the school when the child returns to classes, to ensure that his handling is consistent with his disability. It is not uncommon to find the school restricting the physical activity of a child who is free of any heart disease or real disability, and without any medical recommendation for restriction. On the other hand, when residual disability does exist, the nurse performs an important service in reassuring the patient and his family, explaining the plan of medical care and the long-range outlook, and assisting them in the necessary readjustment. Although primarily designed to benefit the patient, these services also serve as important instruments of continuous community health education.

ROLE OF THE SOCIAL WORKER

The social worker plays an essential part in the comprehensive care of the rheumatic patient. In a long-term study of rheumatic fever at Irvington House (Gavrin et al., 1964) the social worker had three objectives: Primarily, she handled "hard-core" prophylaxis delinquents who could not be induced to attend regularly despite active attempts by physician and nurse. In addition, she provided advice and assistance to patients in paramedical and personal areas related to the illness, for which the medical staff did not have enough time. Finally, in the course of these two activities, the social worker was consulted by many of these families for problems not directly related to the illness, such as housing and employment.

These activities also comprise many of the responsibilities of the social worker in any rheumatic fever clinic. As with many other chronic illnesses, rheumatic fever is the source of considerable parental anxiety relative to genetic factors, chronicity, and life-threatening cardiac damage (Glaser et al., 1961). In her interview, the clinic or hospital social worker tries to uncover the attitude of the patient and family toward the illness and to medical care, and to understand the interrelationships between the patient and other family members. She tries to understand the patient's personality, interests, and anxieties as well as his school achievements and social relationships with his peers. In addition, she gathers information concerning living conditions, income, and related matters which may have great bearing on the long-term care of the patient.

During the acute phase of rheumatic fever the parents require additional support. At this time the social worker can evaluate family stability and other factors which may enable her to recommend whether convalescence should be at home or in a convalescent unit. Her role in rheumatic fever often involves casework with these families. Since rheumatic fever is frequent among people whose income is marginal or below and whose social and economic problems are particularly severe and complex, casework is essential. Rheumatic fever also offers an excellent opportunity for the social worker to engage in group work, with either patients or their families. Such groups are of particular value in convalescent homes for rheumatic fever, where the long-term nature of the disease becomes real to the patient and his parents.

Frequently the social worker may be instrumental in mobilizing a wide variety of community resources—educational, philanthropic, religious, vocational, and so forth. Since physicians and nurses may be unaware of the availability of these services in their community, the social worker serves as an important liaison and resource person in the clinical setting.

FUTURE DIRECTIONS

Methods of rheumatic fever control will undoubtedly change considerably in coming years, and will reflect advances in our understanding of pathogenesis, our technical progress, and the evolution already taking place in the philosophy of our approach to chronic diseases.

Although the close association of the streptococcus and rheumatic fever has been generally accepted for some years, the pathogenetic mechanisms involved continue to elude us. Nevertheless immunization of high-risk groups against streptococcal infections is a definite possibility and an attractive alternative to the cumbersome procedure of long-term antibiotic prophylaxis currently employed. Immunization experiments in animals have been very encouraging (Chapter 14), but considerable work remains before this can become a practical control measure.

Perhaps the most fundamental changes will occur, however, as a result of our evolving philosophy of disease control and prevention. More and more, the community is accepting responsibility for control of diseases that are not contagious and do not represent threats of large-scale epidemics. Increasing public awareness that chronic illness is a great drain on community resources is providing a major stimulus to preventive efforts in many new areas. An income which is marginal or even above that level at normal times may be grossly inadequate for minimal subsistence in times of prolonged illness. By providing the necessary services at critical times for people with such income they may be kept productive and self-supporting, and retain their dignity and self-respect.

The social aspects of rheumatic fever have often been emphasized. The disease is most common among the poorest segment of the population whose members are least able to handle the terrible stresses, financial and otherwise, engendered by long-term illness. Since unemployment is high in this group, and a large part of its working force is unskilled, the vocational handicap produced by rheumatic fever and rheumatic heart disease is particularly significant. In addition, it is a continuing source of concern that although the incidence of rheumatic fever has declined over the past years in the United States as a whole, this downward trend appears to be less striking in areas where poverty prevails.

The long-range attack on streptococcal infections and their rheumatic sequelae therefore involves the improvement of living conditions and in particular the elimination of crowding through improved housing and provision of better nutrition for this segment of our population. The medical services provided must stress continuous preventive care rather than the episodic treatment of acute illness which is often all that is available to those with submarginal incomes. Our overall approach to chronic disease will have to be broadened both in scope and depth. Increased services to a greater number of people will continue to be necessary in coming years. As the battles against acute illness continue to be won, the problems of chronic disease in *all* age groups will demand more and more of the attention of medical and paramedical personnel.

The time-honored boundaries which separate different areas of public health programming today will have to be realigned and at times eliminated. Many of the problems associated with long-term illness are similar regardless of the specific disease involved. At present there is considerable duplication of services by various voluntary agencies dedicated to attacking specific diseases (Hamlin, 1961). Greater integration of their activities, including fund raising, public education, and patient and community services, is essential if unnecessary expenses are to be minimized and if each patient served is to receive the greatest possible benefit.

The punch card and the computer have become part and parcel of the operations of most public health programs. Nevertheless, those who staff these programs must remain constantly aware that services are being rendered to people and not cards, and that human needs must be met. A well functioning and imaginative program must be tempered with the kindness and understanding of those administering it and dispensing its services. Only in this way will program objectives be fully realized in the prevention and control of rheumatic fever and rheumatic heart disease.

This chapter was reviewed by Drs. Arnold Kurlander, Abraham Lillienfeld, Harold Nitowsky, and Jean Stifler. Their critical comments and suggestions are gratefully acknowledged.

Appendices

For the past 25 years the American Heart Association, a voluntary health agency, has played a leading role in establishing programs designed to control heart disease in the United States. Rheumatic fever and rheumatic heart disease have been one of its major interests and this agency has been primarily responsible for the development of prevention programs in this country.

The American Heart Association's Council on Rheumatic Fever and Congenital Heart Disease has prepared and disseminated four important statements designed to assist physicians in the recognition and prevention of rheumatic fever and its complications. These statements have been recently revised and are included as appendices.*

APPENDIX 1.

Jones Criteria (Revised) for Guidance in the Diagnosis of Rheumatic Fever

MAJOR MANIFESTATIONS	MINOR MANIFESTATIONS
Carditis	*Clinical*
Polyarthritis	Fever
Chorea	Arthralgia
Erythema marginatum	Previous rheumatic fever or rheumatic heart disease
Subcutaneous nodules	
	Laboratory
	Acute phase reaction
	Erythrocyte sedimentation rate, C-reactive protein, leukocytosis
	Prolonged PR interval

PLUS

Supporting evidence of preceding streptococcal infection (increased ASO or other streptococcal antibodies; positive throat culture for Group A streptococcus; recent scarlet fever).

The presence of two major criteria, or of one major and two minor criteria, indicates a high probability of the presence of rheumatic fever if supported by evidence of a preceding streptococcal infection. The absence of the latter should make the diagnosis suspect, except in situations in which rheumatic fever is first discovered after a long latent period from the antecedent infection (e.g., Sydenham's chorea or low-grade carditis).

* Courtesy of the American Heart Association.

Rheumatic fever is a sequel to a group A streptococcal infection, but its pathogenesis is unknown. There is no single laboratory test, symptom, or sign which is pathognomonic of the disease, although several *combinations* of them are diagnostic. Various clinical manifestations of rheumatic fever are considered to be part of the same disease because they occur together with a frequency that far exceeds chance.* They may occur singly, however, or in various combinations in any individual patient.

The diagnostic criteria originally proposed by Jones† have proved valuable in preventing overdiagnosis and have been retained. However, some patients present a clinical syndrome which fulfills the original Jones criteria, but which may not be due to rheumatic fever. Acute polyarthritis presents the most common problem. In this revision, therefore, the importance of establishing antecedent streptococcal infection has been emphasized.

The criteria are designed to establish the diagnosis in patients during the acute stage of rheumatic fever. The categories into which clinical and laboratory criteria have been divided are based on the diagnostic importance of a particular finding. They do not relate to prognosis or severity of the disease. They are not a means of measuring rheumatic activity or of establishing the diagnosis of inactive rheumatic heart disease.

The presence of two major criteria, or of one major and two minor criteria, indicates a high probability of the presence of rheumatic fever if supported by evidence of a preceding streptococcal infection. The absence of the latter should always make the diagnosis suspect, except in specific situations described in the section on "Supporting Laboratory Findings." Because the prognosis may differ according to the major manifestations, the diagnosis of rheumatic fever should be followed by a list of the major manifestations present, e.g., rheumatic fever, manifested by polyarthritis and carditis. Also, an indication of the severity of carditis in terms of presence or absence of congestive heart failure and cardiomegaly is advisable.

In addition to the criteria to be used in the recommended formula. other manifestations have been listed which may support the diagnosis. These criteria are not meant to substitute for the judgment of the clinician. They are designed to guide him in the diagnosis of the disease, with the suggestion that he follow questionable cases carefully and restrict diagnosis to illnesses which meet acceptable criteria (see "Overdiagnosis" of Rheumatic Fever).

* By the same token, other streptococcal sequels, typically glomerulonephritis, are not considered part of rheumatic fever because they seldom coexist with polyarthritis, carditis, and so forth.
† Jones, T. D.: Diagnosis of Rheumatic Fever. J.A.M.A. *126*:481-484 (Oct. 21) 1944. These criteria were subsequently modified by a Committee of the American Heart Association in 1955.

MAJOR CLINICAL CRITERIA

Carditis

Rheumatic carditis is almost always associated with a significant murmur. Consequently, the other manifestations listed below, when not associated with a significant murmur, should be labeled carditis with caution.

Murmurs
1. In an individual without previous rheumatic fever or rheumatic heart disease, a significant apical systolic murmur, apical mid-diastolic murmur, or basal diastolic murmur.
2. In an individual with previous rheumatic fever or rheumatic heart disease, a definite change in the character of any of these murmurs or the appearance of a new significant murmur.

Cardiomegaly. Unequivocal cardiac enlargement in an individual without a history of previous rheumatic fever, or an obvious increase in cardiac size in a patient with a past history of rheumatic heart disease.

Pericarditis. Manifested by a friction rub, pericardial effusion, or definite electrocardiographic evidence.

Congestive Heart Failure. In a child or young adult in the absence of other discernible causes.

Polyarthritis

Polyarthritis is almost always migratory and is manifested by swelling, heat, redness, and tenderness, or by pain *and* limitation of motion, of two or more joints. (Arthralgia alone, without other evidence of joint involvement, may occur in rheumatic fever, but is not considered a major manifestation.)

Chorea

Purposeless, involuntary, rapid movements often associated with muscle weakness are characteristic of chorea. These must be differentiated from tics, athetosis, and restlessness. Chorea is a delayed manifestation of rheumatic fever, and other rheumatic manifestations may or may not be present.

Erythema Marginatum

This evanescent, pink rash is characteristic of rheumatic fever. The erythematous areas often have pale centers and round or serpiginous margins. They vary greatly in size and occur mainly on the trunk and proximal part of the extremities, never on the face. The erythema is transient, migrates from place to place, and may be brought out by the application of heat. It is nonpruritic, not indurated, and blanches on pressure.

Subcutaneous Nodules

These firm, painless nodules are seen or felt over the extensor surface of certain joints, particularly elbows, knees, and wrists, in the occipital region, or over the spinous processes of the thoracic and lumbar vertebrae. The skin overlying them moves freely and is not inflamed.

MINOR CRITERIA

Clinical

These are clinical features which occur frequently in rheumatic fever. Because they also occur in many other diseases, their diagnostic value is minor. Their usefulness consists in supporting the diagnosis of rheumatic fever when this diagnosis rests mainly on a single major manifestation.

History of previous rheumatic fever or evidence of pre-existing rheumatic heart disease increases the index of suspicion in evaluating any rheumatic complaint. The history must be well documented, or the evidence of pre-existing rheumatic heart disease clear-cut.

Arthralgia constitutes pain in one or more joints (not in the muscles and other periarticular tissues) without evidence of inflammation, tenderness to touch, or limitation of motion. The presence of arthralgia, in addition to polyarthritis, does not make the latter any more indicative of rheumatic fever, but in the presence of monoarticular arthritis, arthralgia in other joints strengthens the diagnosis of rheumatic fever.

Fever—temperature in excess of 100.4° F. (38° C.) rectally—is usually present early in the course of untreated rheumatic fever.

Laboratory

The acute phase reactants offer objective but nonspecific confirmation of the presence of an inflammatory process. *The erythrocyte sedimentation rate and C-reactive protein test* are most commonly employed. Unless the patient has received corticosteroids or salicylates, these tests are almost always abnormal in patients who present with polyarthritis or acute carditis, whereas they are often normal in patients presenting with chorea. *The erythrocyte sedimentation rate (ESR)* may be markedly increased by anemia and may be decreased in congestive heart failure. *The*

C-reactive protein (CRP) test is a sensitive indicator of inflammation and is negative in uncomplicated anemia. Heart failure due to any cause is often accompanied by a positive CRP test. Sera from normal individuals do not contain this protein, but relatively minor inflammatory stimuli may result in a positive reaction.

Leukocytosis, anemia, or *other non-specific responses* to inflammation may also occur in acute rheumatic fever.

Electrocardiographic changes, mainly PR interval prolongation, are frequent, but may occur in other inflammatory processes. Furthermore, ECG changes that are not associated with clinical evidence of carditis (see Major Clinical Criteria) have a benign prognosis with regard to the ultimate development of rheumatic heart disease. Such changes by themselves, therefore, do not constitute adequate criteria for carditis.

SUPPORTING EVIDENCE OF STREPTOCOCCAL INFECTION

The diagnosis of acute rheumatic fever should never be made solely on the basis of laboratory findings plus minor clinical manifestations. On the other hand, since laboratory indications of recent streptococcal infection and current inflammation occur so regularly with this disease, their unexplained absence should make the physician question the diagnosis of rheumatic fever.

Laboratory Evidence of Preceding Streptococcal Infection—by specific antibody tests or by identification of the offending organism—greatly strengthens the possibility of acute rheumatic fever.

STREPTOCOCCAL ANTIBODY TESTS. The most reliable evidence of a specific infection capable of producing acute rheumatic fever is an increased or, even better, a rising streptococcal antibody titer. These titers differentiate preceding streptococcal from other acute respiratory infections and are increased following asymptomatic as well as symptomatic streptococcal infections.

These antibody levels are generally increased in the early stages of acute rheumatic fever, but may be declining, or low, if the interval from the acute streptococcal infection to the detection of rheumatic fever has been longer than 2 months. This occurs most often in patients whose presenting rheumatic manifestation is chorea. Also, patients whose only major manifestation is rheumatic carditis may have low antibody titers when first seen. Their rheumatic attack may have been in progress several months before becoming symptomatic and thus recognized. Except in the latter two instances, one should be reluctant to make the diagnosis of acute rheumatic fever in the absence of serological evidence of a recent streptococcal infection.

The antistreptolysin O test (ASO) is the most widely used and best standardized streptococcal antibody test. In general, single titers of *at least* 250 Todd units in adults and *at least* 333 units in children over 5 years of age are considered to be increased. Depending on the general prevalence of streptococcal infections, a varying per cent of the normal population may show titers of this magnitude.

About 20 per cent of patients in the early stages of acute rheumatic fever, and most patients who present with chorea, have a low or borderline ASO titer. In these instances, it is advisable to obtain another streptococcal antibody test.* When two or more different streptococcal antibody tests are performed, it is possible to show an increased titer in almost all cases of acute rheumatic fever within the first 2 months of onset, and in about half the cases presenting with chorea. Antibody determination on serum samples obtained at 2 week intervals, preferably performed at the same time, are very useful in documenting a streptococcal infection, especially in patients with very low pre-infection titers. A rise in titers of 2 dilution tubes or more can be demonstrated for at least one of the streptococcal antibodies in almost all recurrent, as well as primary attacks, of rheumatic fever.

ISOLATION OF GROUP A STREPTOCOCCI. Many patients continue to harbor Group A streptococci at the onset of acute rheumatic fever, but these organisms are usually present in small numbers and may be difficult to isolate by a single throat culture. Their demonstration may require special techniques. The administration of penicillin or other antibiotics may also result in failure to isolate the infecting organism. In addition, a significant number of *normal* individuals, particularly children, may harbor Group A streptococci in the upper respiratory tract. For these reasons, throat cultures† are less satisfactory than antibody tests as supporting evidence of recent streptococcal infection.

Clinical Evidence of Preceding Streptococcal Infection. *History of recent attack of scarlet fever* is the best clinical indication of antecedent streptococcal infection.

OTHER CLINICAL FEATURES

These include abdominal pain, rapid sleeping pulse rate (tachycardia out of proportion to fever), malaise, anemia, epistaxis, and precordial pain. They are even more common in other diseases than they are in rheumatic fever, so their usefulness is less than that of the minor criteria.

---

* Available secondary tests include the antihyaluronidase (*ASH*) and antistreptokinase (*ASK*) tests which have been in use for some time, but are difficult to standardize from laboratory to laboratory, and the new antideoxyribonuclease B (anti-DNase B) and anti-diphosphopyridine nucleotidase (anti-DPNase) or antinicotinamide adenine dinucleotidase (anti-NADase) tests which may be easier to standardize.

† A statement entitled "A Method of Culturing Beta Hemolytic Streptococci from the Throat" is included as appendix 4, p. 206.

Although they are not to be considered diagnostic, they provide additional evidence of the presence of rheumatic fever, as does a family history of rheumatic fever.

Combinations of major and minor manifestations and features may be caused by other diseases which may have to be ruled out before a definitive diagnosis of rheumatic fever is made. One combination in particular—polyarthritis, fever, and elevated sedimentation rate—is common in a variety of other disorders. Diseases to be ruled out include rheumatoid arthritis, systemic lupus erythematosus, subacute bacterial endocarditis, serum sickness (including manifestations of penicillin hypersensitivity), gonococcal arthritis, sickle cell anemia, viral pericarditis or myocarditis, leukemia, tuberculosis, undulant fever, and septicemias, particularly meningococcemia. Most of these diseases can be diagnosed with assurance by appropriate tests. Streptococcal antibody determinations are often useful in these differential diagnoses, especially in stimulating the search for other causes when they show no increase.

MURMURS INDICATING CARDITIS

Significant Apical Systolic Murmur (Mitral Regurgitation)

This is a long murmur, filling most of systole. Its blowing quality and high pitch are its most important characteristics. It is heard best in the apical region and is transmitted toward the axilla. The intensity of the murmur is variable, particularly in the early stages of illness, but is at least of grade 2 on a scale of 6. It does not change substantially with position or respiration.

The murmur of mitral regurgitation must be differentiated from functional (innocent) murmurs which frequently occur in normal individuals, especially children. Functional murmurs usually occupy only a portion of systole. They may be quite loud, particularly in anxious or febrile patients, and are rather widely transmitted in thin-chested individuals. These murmurs are heard at times only intermittently and tend to vary with position and respiration. They are usually of two types: an ejection type murmur heard best over the pulmonic area, and a low-pitched, vibratory, groaning or musical murmur heard best along the lower left sternal border. The former is frequently transmitted to the neck and may be mistaken for aortic stenosis. The latter is frequently transmitted to the apex and is most likely to be confused with mitral regurgitation by those unfamiliar with its characteristic quality.

Apical Mid-Diastolic Murmur

Mitral regurgitation and cardiac dilatation accentuate the third heart sound as a result of rapid flow of blood from atrium to ventricle in diastole. During tachycardia, this may produce a protodiastolic gallop rhythm. Frequently, however, in acute rheumatic fever with marked mitral regurgitation, the third heart sound is followed, or replaced, by a low-pitched diastolic rumble. This can be heard best with the patient in the left lateral recumbent position with the breath held in expiration. The same murmur may occur in other forms of acute carditis or in conditions causing rapid blood flow into the left ventricle, such as left to right shunts, hyperthyroidism, sickle cell and other forms of severe anemia. It must be differentiated from the low-pitched, crescendo apical presystolic murmur followed by an accentuated mitral first heart sound, which is indicative of an established mitral stenosis, rather than of acute carditis.

Basal Diastolic Murmur

This murmur of aortic regurgitation begins early in diastole. It is high-pitched, blowing, decrescendo, and is heard best along the left sternal border after deep expiration with the patient leaning forward. It is of great diagnostic importance, but may be difficult to hear and may be present only intermittently.

"OVERDIAGNOSIS" OF RHEUMATIC FEVER

Following a well documented streptococcal infection, the conscientious physician may note suggestive evidence of rheumatic fever, such as vague pains in the extremities, borderline temperature elevations, increased intensity of a functional murmur, tachycardia during the physical examination of an anxious or hyperactive patient, an increased erythrocyte sedimentation rate, and prolonged PR interval in the electrocardiogram. Follow-up of such patients has not revealed the delayed appearance of rheumatic heart disease. In the vast majority of cases, significant murmurs of rheumatic carditis appear within the first few weeks of the disease; very rarely do they appear later than 3 months after the onset of the rheumatic attack, and almost never after 6 months. Patients without significant cardiac murmurs during acute rheumatic fever have an excellent prognosis to escape rheumatic valvular disease.

The diagnosis of acute rheumatic fever should be made, therefore, with conservatism and with insistence upon clearly expressed major clinical manifestations. A common error is the premature, vigorous administration of corticosteroids or salicylates before the signs and symptoms of rheumatic fever are unmistakable. This often leaves an ill-defined syndrome, only presumptively rheumatic fever, and the subsequent management of the patient, particularly the indications for long-term chemoprophylaxis, is in doubt. In the absence of a curative agent, one should not suppress the signs and symptoms of rheumatic fever until they are clearly expressed.

> *AD HOC Committee to revise the Jones Criteria (Modified) of the Council on Rheumatic Fever and Congenital Heart Disease of the American Heart Association*

Gene H. Stollerman, M.D., *Chairman*

Milton Markowitz, M.D.	Lewis W. Wannamaker, M.D.
Angelo Taranta, M.D.	Ruth Whittemore, M.D.

March 5, 1965

APPENDIX 2.

Prevention of Rheumatic Fever

Rheumatic fever is a recurrent disease which frequently can be prevented. Infection with group A streptococci precipitates both initial and recurrent attacks; therefore, prevention of rheumatic fever and rheumatic heart disease depends upon the control of streptococcal infections. This may be accomplished by (1) prevention of streptococcal infections in *rheumatic* subjects, and (2) early and adequate treatment of streptococcal infections in *all* individuals.

Bacterial endocarditis may result from dental and other surgical procedures in patients with rheumatic or congenital heart disease. When such procedures are undertaken, these patients should be protected by *administration of antibiotics in therapeutic doses.**

PREVENTION OF RECURRENCES IN RHEUMATIC INDIVIDUALS

Necessity for Continuous Prophylaxis

Many streptococcal infections occur without producing clinical manifestations. For this reason, prevention of recurrent rheumatic fever must depend on continuous prophylaxis rather than solely on recognition and treatment of acute attacks of streptococcal disease.

General Considerations

Who Should Be Given Prophylaxis?

In general, all patients who have a *well-documented history* of rheumatic fever or chorea, or who show *definite evidence* of rheumatic heart disease, should be given continuous prophylaxis.

How Long Should Prophylaxis Be Continued?

The risk of acquiring a streptococcal infection and the possibility of recurrent attacks of rheumatic fever continue throughout life. It is, therefore, suggested that the *safest general procedure* is to continue prophylaxis indefinitely, particularly if rheumatic heart disease is present.

* A statement entitled "Prevention of Bacterial Endocarditis" is included as appendix 3, p. 203.

Should Exceptions Be Made?

Although recurrent attacks of rheumatic fever occur at any age, the risk of recurrences decreases with the passage of years. Some physicians may wish to make exceptions to instituting or maintaining prophylaxis in certain of their adult patients, particularly those without heart disease who have had no rheumatic attacks for many years. Before exceptions are made, the physician should carefully weigh the risks of acquiring strepto-coccal infection as well as the consequences of recurrence. Individuals with a high risk of exposure to streptococcal infections include young men in military service, mothers of young children, school teachers, and hos-pital nurses.

When Should Prophylactic Treatment Be Initiated?

Prophylaxis should be initiated as soon as the diagnosis of active or inactive rheumatic fever is made.

Patients with rheumatic fever or rheumatic heart disease are often exposed to increased hazards in hospital wards as the result of contact with streptococcal carriers or patients with active streptococcal infections. Care should be taken to avoid interruption or delay in initiating prophy-laxis in hospitalized patients.

Should Prophylaxis Be Continued During the Summer?

Yes, continuously. Streptococcal infections can occur at any season, although they are more prevalent in the winter and spring months.

INITIAL ERADICATION OF RESIDUAL STREPTOCOCCI

Before initiating continuous prophylaxis in patients with active or inactive rheumatic fever, a full therapeutic course of penicillin (as out-lined under Recommended Treatment Schedules, p. 201) should be given to eradicate streptococci which may or may not be detectable by the usual culture techniques.

CHOICE OF PROPHYLACTIC PROGRAM

Several effective methods of continuous prophylaxis are available, and the physician must decide which is most suitable for an individual patient.

Intramuscular vs. Oral Route

The most consistently reliable results have been obtained with intra-muscular benzathine penicillin G. Although many physicians and most patients prefer oral medication, successful oral prophylaxis depends on patient cooperation. Most failures occur in patients who fail to ingest the drug regularly. Patients should receive careful and repeated instructions on this point from the physician. Patients who may be considered unreliable in taking oral medication should receive benzathine penicillin G intramuscularly.

Oral Penicillin vs. Oral Sulfonamides

In the doses recommended sulfadiazine and oral penicillin are equally effective in preventing streptococcal infection and recurrence of rheumatic fever. Although streptococci resistant to sulfonamides have appeared during mass prophylaxis in the armed forces, this is rare in civilian populations. Strains of group A streptococci resistant to penicillin have not been encountered. Patients on penicillin prophylaxis are more likely to harbor staphylococci which are resistant to penicillin, but rarely does this appear to be of clinical significance.

Benzathine Penicillin G—Intramuscular

Dosage—1,200,000 units a month.

Reactions—Some discomfort at the injection site is usual.

Urticaria and angioneurotic edema may occur in a few patients.

Reactions similar to serum sickness include fever and joint pains and may be mistaken for rheumatic fever.

A *careful history of allergic reactions* to penicillin should be obtained. Although many individuals who have had reactions to penicillin may subsequently be able to tolerate the drug, it is safer not to use penicillin if the reaction has been severe and particularly if angioneurotic edema has occurred.

Sulfadiazine—Oral

Dosage—1 Gm. once a day for patients over 60 pounds; 0.5 Gm. for patients under 60 pounds.

Reactions are infrequent and usually minor. In any patient being given sulfonamides, all rashes and sore throats should be investigated as possible reactions, especially if they occur in the first eight weeks.

The chief reactions are:

SKIN ERUPTIONS. Morbilliform—continue drug with caution. Urticaria or scarlatiniform rash associated with sore throat or fever—discontinue drug.

LEUKOPENIA. Discontinue drug if white blood count falls below 4,000 and polynuclear neutrophils fall below 35% because of possible agranulocytosis which is often associated with sore throat and a rash. Because of the possibility of leukopenia developing, weekly white blood counts are advisable for the first two months of prophylaxis. The occurrence of agranulocytosis after eight weeks of continuous prophylaxis with sulfonamides is extremely rare.

Penicillin—Oral

Dosage—200,000 or 250,000 units once or twice a day. Twice daily is probably more effective.

Although other kinds of penicillin may be used, buffered penicillin G is satisfactory. Better blood levels may be obtained if the penicillin is ingested half an hour before or at least one hour after a meal.

Reactions are similar to those with intramuscular penicillin, but occur less frequently and tend to be less severe. A careful history concerning penicillin allergy should, however, be obtained.

TREATMENT OF STREPTOCOCCAL INFECTIONS IN RHEUMATIC INDIVIDUALS

When streptococcal infections occur despite a prophylactic regimen, or occur in a rheumatic subject who is not receiving continuous prophylaxis, they should be treated promptly and vigorously (see the next section). Some physicians may prefer to use injections of 600,000 units of procaine penicillin once or twice daily for 10 days under these circumstances.

Despite optimal therapy, it is sometimes not possible to prevent rheumatic recurrences once streptococcal infections occur in the rheumatic subject.

STREPTOCOCCAL INFECTIONS IN THE GENERAL POPULATION

During epidemics it has been found that about 3% of untreated streptococcal infections are followed by rheumatic fever. Attack rates following sporadic infections are less firmly established. In endemic situations, attack rates may be lower, although it may be more difficult under these circumstances to differentiate infection from the carrier state. Adequate and early penicillin treatment will eliminate streptococci from the throat and prevent most attacks of rheumatic fever.

DIAGNOSIS OF STREPTOCOCCAL INFECTIONS

The accurate recognition of individual streptococcal infections, their adequate treatment, and the control of epidemics in the community presently offer the first practical means of preventing initial attacks of rheumatic fever.

About half of the streptococcal infections which occur are likely to escape detection because they are asymptomatic or atypical. The other half can often be suspected by their clinical manifestations. However, in the absence of a scarlatinal rash, it is impossible to differentiate streptococcal infections with certainty on clinical grounds alone. Therefore, *bacteriological support (by throat culture) of the clinical impression is highly desirable.** The following section on diagnosis has been included in order to assist physicians in making a correct diagnosis and assuring adequate treatment.

Symptoms

Sore throat—sudden onset, pain on swallowing
Headache—common
Fever—variable, but generally from 101° to 104° F.
Abdominal pain—more common in children than in adults
Nausea and vomiting—common, especially in children

Signs

Red throat
Exudate—usually present, may not appear until after the first day
Lymphadenopathy—swollen, *tender* lymph nodes at angle of jaw
Rash—scarlatiniform, when present, usually diagnostic of a streptococcal infection
Acute otitis media ⎫
Acute sinusitis ⎬ may be due to the streptococcus

In the absence of the above symptoms and signs, occurrence of any of the following symptoms is usually *not* associated with a streptococcal infection: simple coryza, hoarseness, cough, conjunctivitis.

Laboratory Findings

Throat culture*—hemolytic streptococci are almost invariably recovered on culture during acute streptococcal infections. A single well-done culture with a quantitative report is usually sufficient, although hemolytic streptococci which are occasionally missed on initial culture may be detected in subsequent cultures.
White blood count—generally over 12,000.

* A statement entitled "A Method for Culturing Beta Hemolytic Streptococci" is included as appendix 4, p. 206.

TREATMENT OF STREPTOCOCCAL INFECTIONS

Treatment should be started as soon as possible, but the short delay entailed in making a diagnosis by awaiting the results of a throat culture does *not* appreciably reduce the efficacy of antibiotic treatment in preventing the occurrence of rheumatic fever. Even when therapy is delayed as long as a week, a significant reduction in the attack rate occurs.

Penicillin is the drug of choice. Continued therapy *for a period of 10 days* is necessary to prevent rheumatic fever, which depends upon eradication of streptococci from the throat. Despite prolonged treatment, streptococci may sometimes fail to be eradicated, especially when oral therapy is used. If possible in patients treated orally, a follow-up culture several days after discontinuing treatment is desirable to ascertain the absence of hemolytic streptococci.

Penicillin may be administered by either the intramuscular or oral route. Administration of the very long-acting repository benzathine penicillin G is recommended as a method of choice since it insures continued treatment for a sufficient length of time. Oral therapy, by contrast, is dependent upon the cooperation of the patient.

RECOMMENDED TREATMENT SCHEDULES

Intramuscular Penicillin

Benzathine penicillin G*
Children—one intramuscular injection of 600,000 to 900,000 units.* (The larger dose is probably preferable for children over 10 years of age.)
Adults—one intramuscular injection of 900,000 to 1,200,000 units.*

Oral Penicillin

Children and adults—200,000 or 250,000 units† three or four times a day for a *full 10 days*. Therapy must be continued for the *entire 10 days* even though the temperature returns to normal and the patient is asymptomatic.

Combined Therapy

Various combinations of oral and intramuscular penicillin should be effective provided adequate coverage is continued for 10 days. For

---

* Mixtures containing shorter acting penicillin should not be substituted for the recommended doses of benzathine penicillin G.

† Of the various oral forms available, buffered penicillin G is satisfactory and less expensive. Although higher blood levels may be achieved with alpha-phenoxymethyl penicillin (penicillin V) or alpha-phenoxyethyl penicillin (phenethicillin), especially when taken near meals, their superiority in the prevention of rheumatic fever has not been documented.

example, one or more injections of procaine penicillin G (600,000 units every 12 to 24 hours) might be followed by oral penicillin for 10 days or an injection of benzathine penicillin G* in recommended doses.

Other Antibiotics

Erythromycin is the most effective antibiotic in patients who are sensitive to penicillin. If given *for 10 days,* this antibiotic is probably as effective as *oral* penicillin in the treatment of streptococcal infections. Although tetracyclines may be effective, a high prevalence of strains resistant to this antibiotic makes it unreliable.

Not Recommended

The sulfonamide drugs should *not* be used for the *treatment* of streptococcal infections. In an established infection, they will not eradicate the streptococcus and therefore will not prevent rheumatic fever. However, the sulfonamides *are* effective in preventing reinfection and recurrences when administered as *continuous prophylaxis* to rheumatic subjects. (See specific prophylactic methods.)

Antibiotic troches and lozenges are also inadequate for the treatment of streptococcal infections because they do not eliminate the streptococcus.

Streptococcal Infections in Contacts

Approximately 25% of household contacts of index cases will contract streptococcal infections, which may vary in degree of severity from asymptomatic disease to frank clinical illness. Therefore, when a well-documented streptococcal infection is found, efforts should be made for detection of infections in other members of the family by a careful history, inspection of the throat and a routine throat culture, when available. Contacts who have manifestations of a respiratory tract infection or large numbers of beta hemolytic streptococci on culture should be treated. Because even delayed therapy will significantly reduce attack rates of rheumatic fever, contacts who have had clinical evidence of a recent streptococcal infection likewise should receive treatment.

This statement was prepared by the Committee on Prevention of Rheumatic Fever and Bacterial Endocarditis of the Council on Rheumatic Fever and Congenital Heart Disease of the American Heart Association:

Lewis W. Wannamaker, M.D., *Chairman*

Floyd W. Denny, M.D.   Maclyn McCarty, M.D.
Antoni Diehl, M.D.   Edward A. Mortimer, M.D.
Ernest Jawetz, M.D.   Philip Y. Paterson, M.D.
Milton Markowitz, M.D.   William Perry, M.D.
Gene H. Stollerman, M.D.

* Mixtures containing shorter acting penicillin should not be substituted for the recommended doses of benzathine penicillin G.

Prevention of Bacterial Endocarditis

In individuals with rheumatic or congenital heart disease, bacteria present in the blood may lodge on damaged heart valves or other parts of the endocardium and cause bacterial endocarditis. For this reason, bacteremia, even though transitory, constitutes a potential threat in such patients.

It is established that transitory bacteremia may result from tooth extraction, oral surgical procedures, manipulation of periodontal tissues, removal of tonsils and adenoids, bronchoscopy, and instrumentation of the genito-urinary tract. Although not as well documented, it is probable that transitory bacteremia may also be associated with other procedures such as cardiac catheterization,* sigmoidoscopy, childbirth, and surgery of the lower intestinal tract.

In patients with rheumatic or congenital heart disease, it is believed that antibiotics should be used in conjunction with the above procedures to decrease the likelihood that bacterial endocarditis will occur. The purpose of using antibiotics is to (1) prevent bacteremia or reduce its magnitude and duration should it occur; and (2) eradicate bacteria that may implant on heart valves before a vegetation is formed.

DENTAL MANIPULATION, ORAL SURGERY, AND BRONCHOSCOPY

Penicillin is the drug of choice. While broad-spectrum antibiotics may decrease bacteremia, they cannot be relied upon to eradicate initial bacterial implants and for this reason are not recommended. Sulfonamides are completely unsatisfactory.

Optimal dosage and duration of therapy with penicillin are not known. It should be emphasized that good evidence exists that penicillin or sulfonamides, in the doses used for prophylaxis against Group A streptococcal infection and consequent recurrence of rheumatic fever, are *not* adequate for prevention of bacterial endocarditis. Larger doses of penicillin are required to prevent implantation of bacteria on heart valves, and a high concentration of penicillin in the blood for several days may well be required to eradicate small bacterial implants should they occur.

* Many cardiologists feel that the low risk of bacterial endocarditis following cardiac catheterization does not justify the routine use of antibiotics in this situation.

It should also be stressed that there is no disagreement concerning the advisability of using *penicillin immediately before and subsequent to the above procedures.* The wisdom of using antibiotics for several days before these procedures are carried out is not yet settled. Such pretreatment with penicillin is not likely to sterilize root abscesses or infected tonsils. Furthermore, some evidence exists that pretreatment may cause sensitive bacteria (e.g., viridans streptococci and staphylococci), normally present in the oral cavity and upper respiratory tract, to be replaced by penicillin-resistant strains. Bacterial endocarditis resulting from such strains would pose greater therapeutic problems.

With the above reservations in mind, the following treatment schedules are suggested:

SUGGESTED TREATMENT SCHEDULES

Day of Procedure. Procaine penicillin 600,000 units supplemented by 600,000 units crystalline penicillin intramuscularly one to two hours before procedure.

    Intramuscular penicillin is more reliable. However, because of practical considerations, some dentists and physicians rely on oral penicillin when the full cooperation of the patient is assured. If oral penicillin is to be employed, four doses (every 4-6 hours) of at least 0.25 Gm. of alpha-phenoxymethyl penicillin (Penicillin V) or 0.25 Gm. of alpha-phenoxyethyl penicillin (phenethicillin), or 500,000 units of buffered penicillin G should be given during the day of the procedure. In addition, an extra dose should be taken one hour before the procedure.

For Two Days After Procedure. Procaine penicillin 600,000 units intramuscularly each day. In selected instances, 0.25 Gm. of alpha-phenoxymethyl penicillin (Penicillin V) or 0.25 Gm. of alpha-phenoxyethyl penicillin (phenethicillin), or 500,000 units of buffered penicillin G four times daily by mouth on each day may be used for those patients in whom full cooperation is anticipated and ingestion is assured.

Contra-indications to Above Regimen. The main contra-indication is sensitivity to penicillin. All patients should be carefully questioned for previous history suggesting penicillin sensitivity. If such a history is obtained, even if equivocal, penicillin should not be given. Under such circumstances, erythromycin should be used in a dose of 250 mg. by mouth four times daily for adults and older children. For small children, a dose of 20 mg. per pound per day divided into three or four evenly spaced doses may be used. The total dose should not exceed 1 Gm. per day.

INSTRUMENTATION OF GENITO-URINARY TRACT, SURGERY OF THE LOWER INTESTINAL TRACT, AND CHILDBIRTH

With these procedures, transitory bacteremia due to penicillin-resistant enterococci is apt to occur. The use of penicillin alone in the doses as suggested above cannot be expected to curtail bacteremia due to enterococci, a common cause of bacterial endocarditis.

For these reasons, it is suggested that as an empirical guide, the above intramuscular penicillin regimen be used in combination with streptomycin 1 or 2 Gm. intramuscularly on the day of procedure and for each of two days following the procedure. In children, streptomycin may be given in a dosage of 50 mg./kg., not to exceed 1 Gm. per day. In patients who are sensitive to penicillin, a combination of erythromycin and streptomycin or a broad-spectrum antibiotic combined with streptomycin may be of some use, although it should be emphasized that very little information is available about these antibiotic combinations and their efficacy in preventing bacterial endocarditis due to enterococci.

This statement was prepared by the Committee on Prevention of Rheumatic Fever and Bacterial Endocarditis of the Council on Rheumatic Fever and Congenital Heart Disease of the American Heart Association

Lewis W. Wannamaker, M.D., *Chairman*

Floyd W. Denny, M.D.	Maclyn McCarty, M.D.
Antoni Diehl, M.D.	Edward A. Mortimer, M.D.
Ernest Jawetz, M.D.	Philip Y. Paterson, M.D.
William M. M. Kirby, M.D.	William Perry, M.D.
Milton Markowitz, M.D.	Charles H. Rammelkamp, Jr., M.D.

Gene H. Stollerman, M.D.

APPENDIX 4.

A Method for Culturing Beta Hemolytic
Streptococci From the Throat

THE VALUE OF THROAT CULTURES TO THE
PRACTICING PHYSICIAN

Except in the case of scarlet fever, no completely satisfactory clinical criteria are available for distinguishing patients with streptococcal respiratory infections from those with respiratory illnesses due to other agents. Many instances of pharyngitis and tonsillitis—with or without exudate—are non-bacterial in etiology; some have been linked with the new group of adenoviruses. These non-streptococcal infections do not lead to rheumatic fever, and patients with such infections are not benefited by antibiotic therapy.

Because the diagnosis of a streptococcal infection of the upper respiratory tract on clinical grounds is necessarily presumptive, a culture of the throat provides valuable laboratory confirmation or rejection of the clinical impression. Throat cultures from patients with acute streptococcal infections are positive for beta hemolytic streptococci in over 95 per cent of cases.

A throat culture is a relatively simple laboratory procedure to perform, and a preliminary report is available within 18 hours. In certain doubtful cases, it is possible for the physician to use his judgment in withholding antibiotic therapy until the results of the throat culture are available. A throat culture is also a useful guide for determining whether treatment with penicillin need be continued for the full ten days recommended for bona fide streptococcal infections. Compared with many other laboratory diagnostic aids, a throat culture is nominal in cost. The cost may be more than redeemed by the savings from withholding or discontinuing useless antibiotic therapy.

As with other laboratory tests, a throat culture may be misleading unless properly taken, processed, and interpreted. For example, a common error is to confuse the non-pathogenic green (alpha) streptococci with those which produce upper respiratory infections. It is therefore essential that the practicing physician have some knowledge of the entire procedure, both to insure that the culture is correctly taken and handled, and to evaluate the reports received from the laboratory.

Many techniques have been employed for the isolation of beta hemolytic streptococci, and a more detailed discussion of the problem may be found elsewhere. The object here is to present briefly a simple method which has proved successful in identifying these organisms in cultures of the throat.

PREPARATION OF MEDIA

A suitable medium for identifying beta hemolytic streptococci should be prepared *before the throat culture is taken* in order to avoid delay in inoculation. Beta hemolytic streptococci are most easily identified on sheep blood agar plates.

Sheep blood* is collected aseptically by venipuncture and defibrinated by slow rotation for approximately ten minutes in a flask containing glass beads. Blood may be stored at refrigerator temperatures for one or two weeks but should be checked for contamination and hemolysis before use. Preservatives should be avoided, as these may inhibit growth on the final culture medium.

A commercially available blood agar base† is prepared and sterilized according to directions. If, after sterilizing, the agar base is allowed to harden, it must be thoroughly reheated in a boiling water bath to remove lumps. The heated agar is cooled to 45-50° C. A constant temperature bath is convenient for achieving and maintaining this temperature, but with experience, the proper temperature can be judged by touch. Defibrinated sheep blood to a volume of 5 per cent‡ is added and mixed by gentle rotation. The blood agar mixture is poured into sterile glass or plastic Petri dishes in about 15-20 cc. amounts. The layer of blood agar should be about 6 mm. thick. It is difficult to differentiate the kinds of hemolysis on plates which are either too thin or too thick. A 10 cm. filter-paper disk may be placed in the top of the Petri dish to absorb excess condensed moisture.

Sterile blood agar plates may be stored at room temperature for several days or in the refrigerator for one to two weeks, but with prolonged storage care must be taken to preserve sufficient moisture by sealing with parafilm strips. Plates showing evidence of contamination or hemolysis on storage should be discarded.

---

* Sheep blood is preferable to rabbit, horse, or human blood. Beta hemolytic streptococci are readily differentiated from alpha hemolytic (green) streptococci on sheep blood plates. Sheep blood also contains a factor which inhibits the growth of *Hemophilus hemolyticus*, the colonies of which may be mistaken for those of beta hemolytic streptococci.

† Baltimore Biological Laboratory, Inc., Baltimore 18, Maryland; Colab Laboratories, Chicago Heights, Ill. (Oxoid medium); Difco Laboratories, Detroit, Michigan.

‡ If the hematocrit of the sheep blood is low, 7 to 10 per cent blood may be necessary to obtain satisfactory plates.

Although readily prepared in the hospital or office laboratory, sheep blood agar plates may also be obtained commercially.

TECHNIQUE OF OBTAINING THROAT CULTURE

In order to insure reliable results, throat cultures should be taken before antibiotic therapy is initiated. Failure to isolate beta hemolytic streptococci may also result from faulty technique in obtaining and handling cultures before they reach the laboratory.

Small cotton or Dacron swabs on 2 × 150 mm. sticks are sterilized in individual cotton-plugged test tubes. An adequate culture of the throat cannot be obtained blindly. The tongue should be depressed and the throat adequately exposed and illuminated. Routinely, the swab should be rubbed over each tonsillar area and the posterior pharynx. Any area exhibiting exudate should also be touched. Care should be taken to avoid contaminating the swab by touching the tongue and lips.

The swab is returned to the test tube, labeled, and inoculated onto a blood agar plate as soon as possible. No more than one or two hours should elapse before plates are inoculated. If a longer delay is inevitable, drying may be prevented by placing the swab in a test tube containing 0.5 ml. of broth. The broth-tube method has the disadvantage of permitting overgrowth by other organisms and of interfering with an estimation of the number of beta hemolytic streptococci present.

In order to facilitate prompt inoculation of plates, some physicians keep a stock of blood agar plates in their office and carry a few in their examining bags. For this purpose plates made of disposable plastics and sealed with scotch tape are particularly desirable. A convenient disposable sterile wire loop for immediate streaking of the blood agar plate can be incorporated in the test tube or in a sealed paper envelope along with the sterile throat swab. A partially unbent paper clip sterilized in a match flame may also serve as a handy substitute for a streaking loop.

Other procedures for handling throat swabs, including mail-in procedures, are being used and evaluated in certain communities.

TECHNIQUE OF STREAKING PLATE

The objectives in streaking a blood agar plate are to avoid drying of specimen by delay, to insure adequate distribution so that well-isolated colonies will be present for examination, and to provide for observation of subsurface as well as surface hemolysis.

Upon arrival in the laboratory, the swab should be immediately processed by rubbing and twisting onto the edge of a moist sheep blood agar plate. This initial inoculation with the swab should cover only *about one sixth of the plate*. (The area of inoculation with the swab should not be too large since growth on this area is usually too thick for proper identification.) A sterile wire loop* is streaked through the primary inoculum onto about one half of the plate in 10 to 20 to-and-fro strokes. Without re-entering the site of primary inoculation, the loop is streaked through this area of secondary inoculation onto the remainder of the plate. Finally, several stabs are made into the agar for observation of subsurface hemolysis.† Reheating of the loop is not necessary at any stage of the streaking or stabbing of the plate (see diagram).

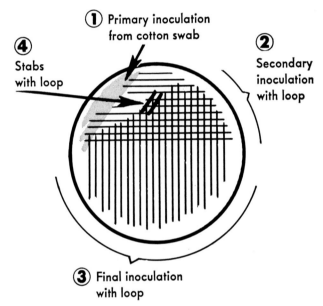

① Primary inoculation from cotton swab

④ Stabs with loop

② Secondary inoculation with loop

③ Final inoculation with loop

Diagram of technique of inoculating and streaking blood agar plate

Inoculated plates are incubated overnight at 37° C. Satisfactory small incubators can be inexpensively constructed or purchased commercially.

TECHNIQUE OF READING PLATE

Streptococci causing acute respiratory infections (beta hemolytic streptococci) are recognized by the clear zone of hemolysis surrounding

* Loops may be sterilized by heating in a flame just prior to using or may be packaged sterilely.
† As an alternative method for observing subsurface (or anaerobic) hemolysis, some laboratories employ pour plates (inoculum incorporated into the blood agar) or anaerobic incubation of surface-inoculated plates.

the colonies. In general, streptococci surrounded by no hemolysis (gamma streptococci) or by green or partial hemolysis (alpha streptococci) are nonpathogenic inhabitants of the throat. Cultures from normal throats usually show numerous streptococci (or sometimes pneumococci) which produce such partial or green hemolysis, and care must be taken not to confuse these with the beta hemolytic streptococci, which cause infections of the throat. This important differentiation may be difficult to make if blood agar plates are too thin or too thick, if growth is too heavy, or if plates are incubated more than 24 hours (e.g., over a week end).

Occasionally, streptococci causing respiratory infections produce partial or green hemolysis on the surface and clear hemolysis in the sub-surface (or stab) growth.

Other organisms which may produce clear hemolysis on sheep blood agar are *hemolytic staphylococci and gram-negative cocci*. To the experienced eye, the appearance of the colony can be helpful, but a Gram stain should be done in all doubtful instances. Chaining of streptococci is more likely to be observed on smears made from broth cultures. On smears made from blood agar plates, it is sometimes difficult to distinguish staphylococci from streptococci. The differentiation may be made by the catalase test.* On horse, rabbit, or human blood agar, *Hemophilus hemolyticus* may closely resemble hemolytic streptococci, but staining reveals gram-negative rods rather than gram-positive cocci in chains.

A complete laboratory report should indicate the relative number of colonies of beta hemolytic streptococci present as well as the kind of hemolysis.

FURTHER LABORATORY CONFIRMATION

Final determination of the kind of hemolysis sometimes cannot be made on the original plate. In such instances, the organism should be isolated in pure culture for further study of the colony formation and of the surface and subsurface (stab) hemolysis.

The procedure outlined does not differentiate between the various groups of beta hemolytic streptococci. Since most strains causing upper respiratory infections in man and all those resulting in rheumatic fever belong to *group A*, identification of the serological group can be of importance in determining whether the full ten-day treatment with penicillin is required. Therefore, it is recommended that whenever possible it should be established whether the organism isolated is group A.

* Add a small amount of growth from blood agar plate to 0.5 cc. of 3 per cent hydrogen peroxide solution. If bubbles of gas appear, the organism is not a streptococcus. Care must be taken not to transfer any of the red blood cells of the medium, because this may give a false positive test. A more reliable test can be obtained on cultures grown on nutrient or serum agar without blood.

The conventional method of determining the serological group is by precipitin test, using a hot acid extract of the bacterial cells and specific grouping antisera.* Several alternate methods are now available, including the use of a *Streptomyces albus* enzyme.†

One of the simplest methods of differentiating group A streptococci is by their bacitracin sensitivity. Colonies of beta hemolytic streptococci are subcultured onto blood agar plates, and a bacitracin-containing paper strip or disk is placed over the area of inoculation so as to influence both heavily and lightly inoculated zones. After 18 to 24 hours' incubation, plates are examined for bacitracin inhibition. If any colonies grow up to the edge of the disk, the strain is recorded as resistant, i.e., non-group A. If inhibition of hemolysis but not of growth is observed, it must be ascertained that the subculture is not a mixture of a sensitive group A strain and a resistant non-beta hemolytic strain. In cases of acute infection, growth of beta hemolytic streptococci may be sufficiently heavy to make a dependable interpretation of inhibition, or lack of inhibition, around a bacitracin disk placed on the primary blood agar plate.

The bacitracin method correlates well with serological grouping when special differentiation disks containing 1-2 units of bacitracin‡ are used, but an appreciable number of false positive results will be obtained if commercial disks designed for routine antibiotic sensitivity screening, which may contain larger quantities of bacitracin, are employed. The use of old disks may produce false negative results. For these reasons it is advisable to include control strains of known bacitracin sensitivity. It should be emphasized that the bacitracin test *only applies to beta hemolytic streptococci.*

Fluorescent antibody§ may be used to identify group A streptococci on smears made from beta hemolytic colonies picked from blood agar plates or on smears made from original throat swabs incubated in broth for 4 hours. Although results are somewhat delayed, the former method appears to be preferable for general purposes since valuable quantitative information is obtained from the conventional blood agar plates and since it avoids tedious screening of many negative cultures with the fluorescent microscope.

By additional serological techniques, group A strains can be subdivided into some 50 different types,‖ but classification according to

* Group A antiserum is now commercially available (Baltimore Biological Laboratories; Difco Laboratories). For methods, see Swift, H. F.: The Streptococci. In Bacterial and Mycotic Infections of Man. Dubos, R. J., ed. J. B. Lippincott Company, Philadelphia, 1948, p. 237.
† Commercially available (Difco Laboratories).
‡ Commercially available (Baltimore Biological Laboratories; Difco Laboratories).
§ Commercially available (Difco Laboratories; Sylvana Chemical Co., Orange, New Jersey).
‖ Typing antisera are not commercially available.

specific types is ordinarily beyond the interests or needs of the routine diagnostic laboratory.

CLINICAL INTERPRETATION OF LABORATORY REPORTS

With the simple precautions outlined above, it is rare that beta hemolytic streptococci are missed on throat cultures obtained from active untreated streptococcal infections. Negative cultures are often obtained on patients in whom treatment has been initiated. Only a few hours of antibiotic therapy may result in suppression of the organism so that isolation becomes difficult or impossible.

In active, untreated streptococcal infections, colonies of beta hemolytic streptococci are often present in large numbers on the blood agar plate. The beta hemolytic streptococcus is usually the predominant organism. Quantitation is therefore an important aspect of culture reports.

It should be borne in mind that the isolation of beta hemolytic streptococci does not necessarily indicate active streptococcal infection. A significant number of normal individuals harbor beta hemolytic streptococci which may be incorrectly accepted as the etiological agent when isolated during the course of a non-streptococcal respiratory infection. In such chronic carriers, only a few colonies of beta hemolytic streptococci are usually found and these may be non-group A (i.e., not associated with rheumatic fever). In interpreting the laboratory report, attention should be paid to the number of colonies of beta hemolytic streptococci present and the serological group should be obtained whenever possible. In all instances, the laboratory results should be considered in conjunction with clinical and epidemiological evidence in order to arrive at the most reasonable diagnosis.

Additional evidence of active streptococcal infection may be obtained by streptococcal antibody studies; e.g., antistreptolysin O or ASO titers, on patients' sera. These are not commonly obtained except in epidemiological studies or in patients with suspected complications of streptococcal infection (acute rheumatic fever or acute nephritis).

This statement was prepared by Lewis W. Wannamaker, M.D., at the request of the Committee on Prevention of Rheumatic Fever and Bacterial Endocarditis of the Council on Rheumatic Fever and Congenital Heart Disease.

REFERENCES

Adams, S. S. and Cobb, R.: The effect of salicylates and related compounds on erythema in the guinea-pig and man. *In*: Salicylates, An International Symposium, page 127. Ed. Dixon, A. St. J.; Martin, B. K.; Wood, P. H. N.; Smith, M. J. H. Little, Brown and Co., Boston, 1963.

Ainger, L. E.; Ely, R. S.; Done, A. K.; and Kelley, V. C.: Sydenham's chorea. II. Effects of hormone therapy. Amer. J. Dis. Child. 89:580, 1955.

Alexander, W. D. and Smith, G.: Disadvantageous circulatory effects of salicylate in rheumatic fever. Lancet 1:768, 1962.

Alimurung, M. M. and Massell, B. F.: The normal P-R interval in infants and children. Circulation 13:257, 1956.

Ambuel, J. P.; Cebulla, J.; Watt, N.; and Crowne, D. P.: Urgency as a factor in clinic attendance. Amer. J. Dis. Child. 108:394, 1964.

Anderson, H. C.; Kunkel, H. G.; and McCarty, M.: Quantitative anti-streptokinase studies in patients infected with group A hemolytic streptococci: A comparison with serum antistreptolysin and gamma globulin levels with special reference to the occurrence of rheumatic fever. J. Clin. Invest. 27:425, 1948.

Anderson, H. C. and McCarty, M.: Determination of C-reactive protein in the blood as a measure of the activity of the disease process in acute rheumatic fever. Amer. J. Med. 8:445, 1950.

Angelino, P. F; Levi, V.; Brusca, A.; and Actis-Dato, A.: Mitral commissurotomy in the younger age group. Amer. Heart J. 51:916, 1956.

Arevalo, A. C.; Spagnuolo, M.; and Feinstein, A. R.: A simple electrocardiographic indication of left atrial enlargement. A study of young patients with rheumatic heart disease. J.A.M.A. 185:358, 1963.

Aronson, N.; Douglas, H. S.; and Lewis, J. M.: Cortisone in Sydenham's chorea. J.A.M.A. 145:30, 1951.

Ash, R.: Influence of tonsillectomy on rheumatic infection. Amer. J. Dis. Child. 55:63, 1938.

Ash, R.: The first 10 years of rheumatic infection in childhood. Amer. Heart J. 36:89, 1948.

Ashman, R. and Hull, E.: Essentials of Electrocardiography, for the Student and Practitioner of Medicine. 2nd ed. The Macmillan Co., New York, 1941.

Ayoub, E. M. and Wannamaker, L. W.: Evaluation of the streptococcal desoxyribonuclease B and diphosphopyridine nucleotidase antibody tests in acute rheumatic fever and acute glomerulonephritis. Pediatrics 29:527, 1962.

Baldwin, J. S.: Sulfadiazine prophylaxis in children and adolescents with inactive rheumatic fever. J. Pediat. 30:284, 1947.

Baldwin, J. S.; Kerr, J. M.; Kuttner, A. G.; and Doyle, E. F.: Observations on rheumatic nodules over a 30-year period. J. Pediat. 56:465, 1960.

213

Barkulis, S. S.; Walsh, G.; and Ekstedt, R. D.: Studies of streptococcal cell walls. II. Type-specific antigenicity in rabbits. J. Bact. 76:109, 1958.

Barlow, J. B.; Pocock, W. A.; Marchand, P.; and Denny, M.: The significance of late systolic murmurs. Amer. Heart J. 66:443, 1963.

Barnes, A. R.; Smith, H. L.; Slocumb, C. H.; Polley, H. F.; and Hench, P. S.: Effect of cortisone and corticotropin (ACTH) on the acute phase of rheumatic fever. Further observations. A.M.A. Amer. J. Dis. Child. 82:397, 1951.

Bergman, A. B. and Werner, R. J.: Failure of children to receive penicillin by mouth. New Eng. J. Med. 268:1334, 1963.

Bernhard, G. C. and Stollerman, G. H.: Serum inhibition of streptococcal diphosphopyridine nucleotidase in uncomplicated streptococcal pharyngitis and in rheumatic fever. J. Clin. Invest. 38:1942, 1959.

Bernstein, S. H. and Allerhand, J.: Studies of hypergammaglobulinemia in acute rheumatic fever. Circulation 26:688, 1962.

Bernstein, S. H.; Feldman, H. A.; Harper, O. F.; and Klingensmith, W. H.: Mass oral penicillin prophylaxis in control of streptococcal disease. Arch. Intern. Med. 93:894, 1954.

Bjork, U. O.; Lodin, H.; and Malers, E.: Evaluation of the degree of mitral insufficiency by selective left ventricular angiocardiography. Amer. Heart J. 60:691, 1960.

Blackman, N. S.: Rheumatic fever: the problem of diagnosis based on insufficient evidence. Pediatrics 31:969, 1963.

Bland, E. F.: Chorea as a manifestation of rheumatic fever: A long-term perspective. Trans. Amer. Clin. Climat. Ass. 73:209, 1961.

Bland, E. F. and Jones, T. D.: Rheumatic fever and rheumatic heart disease: A twenty year report on 1000 patients followed since childhood. Circulation 4:836, 1951.

Blumenthal, S.; Griffiths, S. P.; and Morgan, B. C.: Bacterial endocarditis in children with heart disease. A review based on the literature and experience with 58 cases. Pediatrics 26:993, 1960.

Borman, J. B.; Stern, S.; Shapira, T.; Milwidsky, H.; and Braun, K.: Mitral valvotomy in children. Amer. Heart J. 61:763, 1961.

Brand-Auraban, A.: The epidemiology of rheumatic fever in Israel. Harefuah 57:53, 1959 (Heb.).

Branscome, W. C.; Mather, J. A.; Benson, W. W.: Analysis of Idaho case registry for rheumatic fever. Public Health Rep. 78:489, 1963.

Breese, B. B. and Disney, F. A.: Accuracy of diagnosis of beta streptococcal infection on clinical grounds. J. Pediat. 44:670, 1954.

Breese, B. B. and Disney, F. A.: Factors influencing spread of beta hemolytic streptococcal infections within family group. Pediatrics 17:834, 1956.

Breese, B. B. and Disney, F. A.: Penicillin in the treatment of streptococcal infections. A comparison of effectiveness of five different oral and one parenteral form. New Eng. J. Med. 259:57, 1958.

Brest, A. N.; Uricchia, J.; and Likoff, W.: Valvular surgery in the young patient with rheumatic heart disease. J.A.M.A. 171:249, 1959.

Brick, M.; McKinley, H.; Roy, T. E.; and Keith, J. D.: Oral penicillin prophylaxis in rheumatic fever patients. Canad. Med. Ass. J. 63:255, 1950.

Brock, R. C.: The surgical and pathological anatomy of the mitral valve. Brit. Heart J. 14:489, 1952.

Brown, G.; Goldring, D.; and Behrer, M. R.: Rheumatic pneumonia. J. Pediat. 52:598, 1958.

Brownell, K. D. and Stix, R. K.: A public health program for children with heart disease or rheumatic fever. Amer. J. Public Health 53:1587, 1963.

Brumfitt, W.; O'Grady, F.; and Slater, J. D. H.: Benign streptococcal sore throat. Lancet 2:419, 1959.

Buchanan, D. N.: Pathologic changes in chorea. Amer. J. Dis. Child. 62:443, 1941.

Buchanan, D. N.; Walker, A. E.; and Case, T. J.: The pathogenesis of chorea. J. Pediat. 20:555, 1942.

Bunn, W. H. and Bennett, H. N.: Community control of rheumatic fever. J.A.M.A. 157:986, 1955.

Burke, J. B.: Erythema marginatum. Arch. Dis. Child. *30*:359, 1955.

Burke, P. J.: Penicillin prophylaxis in acute rheumatism. Lancet *1*:255, 1947.

Bywaters, E. G. L.: The relation between heart and joint disease including "rheumatoid heart disease" and chronic post-rheumatic arthritis (type Jaccoud). Brit. Heart J. *12*:101, 1950.

Bywaters, E. G. L. and Thomas, G. T.: Bed rest, salicylates and steroid in rheumatic fever. Brit. Med. J. *1*:1628, 1961.

Cabrera, E. C. and Monray, J. R.: Systolic and diastolic loading of the heart. II. Electrocardiographic data. Amer. Heart J. *43*:669, 1952.

Caceres, C. A.; Steinberg, C. A.; Abraham, S.; Carbery, W. J.; McBride, J. M.; Tolles, W. E.; and Rikli, A. E.: Computer extraction of electrocardiographic parameters. Circulation *25*:356, 1962.

Caffey, J.: Pediatric X-ray Diagnosis. Year Book Medical Publishers, Inc., Chicago, 1950.

Cahan, J. M.: Rheumatic heart disease in Philadelphia school children. Ann. Intern. Med. *10*:1752, 1937.

Carlson, A. S.; Kellner, A.; Bernheimer, A. W.; and Freeman, E. B.: A streptococcal enzyme that acts specifically upon diphosphopyridine nucleotide. J. Exp. Med. *106*:15, 1957.

Carmichael, D. B.: The corrected Q-T duration in acute convalescent rheumatic fever. Amer. Heart J. *50*:528, 1955.

Carter, M. E.; Bywaters, E. G. L.; and Thomas, G. T. G.: Rheumatic fever treated with penicillin in bactericidal dosage for six weeks. Report of a small controlled trial. Brit. Med. J. *1*:965, 1962.

Castle, R. F. and Baylin, G. J.: Severe acquired mitral stenosis in childhood and adolescence. J. Pediat. *58*:404, 1961.

Catanzaro, F. J.; Brock, L.; Chamovitz, R.; Perry, W. D.; Siegel, A. C.; Stetson, C. A.; Rammelkamp, C. H.; Houser, H. B.; Stolzer, B. L.; Wannamaker, L. W.; and Hahn, E. O.: Effect of the oxytetracycline therapy of streptococcal sore throat on the incidence of acute rheumatic fever. Ann. Intern. Med. *42*:345, 1955.

Catanzaro, F. J.; Rammelkamp, C. H.; and Chamovitz, R.: Prevention of rheumatic fever by treatment of streptococcal infection. II. Factors responsible for failure. New Eng. J. Med. *259*:51, 1958.

Catanzaro, F. J.; Stetson, C. A.; Morris, A. J.; Chamovitz, R.; Rammelkamp, C. H., Jr.; Stolzer, B. L.; and Perry, W. D.: The role of the streptococcus in the pathogenesis of rheumatic fever. Amer. J. Med. *17*:749, 1954.

Chamovitz, R.; Catanzaro, F. J.; Stetson, C. A.; and Rammelkamp, C. H., Jr.: Prevention of rheumatic fever by treatment of previous streptococcal infections. I. Evaluation of benzathine penicillin G. New Eng. J. Med. *251*:466, 1954.

Chamovitz, R.; Rammelkamp, C. H., Jr.; Wannamaker, L. W.; and Denny, F. W., Jr.: The effect of tonsillectomy on the incidence of streptococcal respiratory disease and its complications. Pediatrics *26*:355, 1960.

Chandler, C. A. and Taussig, H. B.: Sulfanilamide as a prophylactic agent in rheumatic fever. Bull. Johns Hopkins Hosp. *72*:42, 1943.

Chapman, A. H.; Pilkey, L.; and Gibbons, M. J.: A psychosomatic study of eight children with Sydenham's chorea. Pediatrics *21*:582, 1958.

Chavez, I.: The incidence of heart disease in Mexico; study of 2400 cases of organic heart disease. Amer. Heart J. *24*:88, 1942.

Cheadle, W. B.: Harveian lectures on the various manifestations of the rheumatic state as exemplified in childhood and early life. Lancet *1*:821, 871, 921, 1889.

Cheadle, W. B.: The Various Manifestations of the Rheumatic State as Exemplified in Childhood and Early Life. Smith, Elder and Co., London, 1889.

Clarke, C. A.; McConnell, R. B.; and Sheppard, P. M.: ABO blood groups and secretor character in rheumatic carditis. Brit. Med. J. *1*:21, 1960.

Clarke, P. J. H.: Clinical and public health aspects of juvenile rheumatism in Dublin. Irish J. Med. Sci. pp. 97-118, March, 1940.

Coburn, A. F.: The continuous association of poverty with intensity of rheumatic manifestations. Amer. J. Med. Sci. *240*:687, 1960.

Coburn, A. F.: The Factor of Infection in the Rheumatic State. Williams and Wilkins Co., Baltimore, 1931.

Coburn, A. F.: Salicylate therapy in rheumatic fever: A rational technique. Bull. Johns Hopkins Hosp. 73:435, 1943.

Coburn, A. F. and Moore, L. V.: The independence of chorea and rheumatic activity. Amer. J. Med. Sci. 193:1, 1937.

Coburn, A. F. and Moore, L. V.: The prophylactic use of sulfanilamide in streptococcal respiratory infections with especial reference to rheumatic fever. J. Clin. Invest. 18:147, 1939.

Coburn, A. F. and Pauli, R. H.: Active and passive immunization to hemolytic streptococcus in relation to the rheumatic process. J. Clin. Invest. 14:763, 1935.

Coburn, A. F. and Young, D. C.: The epidemiology of hemolytic streptococcus during World War II in the United States Navy. Williams and Wilkins Co., Baltimore, 1949.

Cochran, J. B.: The anaemia of rheumatic fever. Brit. Med. J. 2:637, 1951.

Cole, L. R.: Cardiac disease among 28,139 newly entering students at the University of Wisconsin. Amer. J. Med. Sci. 201:197, 1941.

Collier, H. O. J.: Antagonism by aspirin and like-acting drugs in kinins and SRS-A in guinea-pig lung. In: Salicylates, An International Symposium, page 120. Ed. Dixon, A. St. J.; Martin, B. K.; Wood, P. H. N.; and Smith, M. J. H. Little, Brown and Co., Boston, 1963.

Collins, S. D.: The incidence of rheumatic fever as recorded in general morbidity surveys of families. Public Health Rep. Suppl. 198, 1947.

Collis, W. R. F.: Acute rheumatism and haemolytic streptococci. Lancet 1:1341, 1931.

Collis, W. R. F.: Bacteriology of rheumatic fever. Lancet 2:817, 1939.

Collis, W. R. F. and Sheldon, W.: Intravenous vaccines of haemolytic streptococci in acute rheumatism in childhood. Lancet 2:1261, 1932.

Combined Rheumatic Fever Study Group, 1960: A comparison of the effect of prednisone and acetylsalicylic acid on the incidence of residual rheumatic heart disease. New Eng. J. Med. 262:895, 1960.

Combined Rheumatic Fever Study Group, 1965: A comparison of short-term, intensive prednisone and acetylsalicylic acid therapy in the treatment of acute rheumatic fever. New Eng. J. Med. 272:63, 1965.

Commission on Acute Respiratory Diseases. Fort Bragg, N. C.: A study of a foodborne epidemic of tonsillitis and pharyngitis due to B-hemolytic streptococcus, type 5. Bull. Johns Hopkins Hosp. 77:143, 1945.

Coombs, C. F.: Rheumatic Heart Disease. William Wood and Co., New York, 1924.

Cornfeld, D.; Werner, G.; Weaver, R.; Bellows, M. T.; and Hubbard, J. P.: Streptococcal infection in a school population: Preliminary report. Ann. Intern. Med. 49:1305, 1958.

Cromartie, W. J.: Reactions of connective tissue to cellular components of group A streptococci. In: The Streptococcus, Rheumatic Fever and Glomerulonephritis, page 187. Ed. Uhr, J. W. Williams and Wilkins Co., Baltimore, 1964.

Cutler, J. G.; Ongley, P. A.; Shwachman, H.; Massell, B. F.; and Nadas, A. S.: Bacterial endocarditis in children with heart disease. Pediatrics 22:706, 1958.

Czoniczer, G.; Amezuca, F.; Pelargonio, S.; and Massell, B. F.: Therapy of severe rheumatic carditis: Comparison of adrenocortical steroids and aspirin. Circulation 29:813, 1964.

Czoniczer, G.; Lees, M.; and Massell, B. F.: Streptococcal infection: The need for improved recognition and treatment for the prevention of rheumatic fever. New Eng. J. Med. 265:951, 1961.

Dack, S.; Bleifer, S.; Grishman, A.; and Donoso, E.: Mitral stenosis; auscultatory and phonocardiographic findings. Amer. J. Cardiol. 5:815, 1960.

Damrosch, D. S.: Chemoprophylaxis and sulfonamide resistant streptococci. J.A.M.A. 130:124, 1946.

Daugherty, S. C. and Schmidt, W. C.: Current considerations regarding the prevention of primary and recurrent rheumatic fever. Med. Clin. N. Amer. 47:1301, 1963.

Davies, A. M. and Lazarov, E.: Heredity, infection and chemoprophylaxis in rheumatic carditis: An epidemiologic study of a communal settlement. J. Hyg. (Camb.) 58:263, 1960.

Davis, J. and Schmidt, W. C.: Benzathine penicillin G: Its effectiveness in the prevention of streptococcal infections in a heavily exposed population. New Eng. J. Med. 256:339, 1957.

Decker, J. P.; Hawn, C. VanZ.; and Robbins, S. L.: Rheumatic "activity" as judged by the presence of Aschoff bodies in auricular appendages of patients with mitral stenosis. I. Anatomical aspects. Circulation 8:161, 1953.

Denny, F. W., Jr.; Perry, W. D.; and Wannamaker, L. W.: Type-specific streptococcal antibody. J. Clin. Invest. 36:1092, 1957.

Denny, F. W., Jr.; Wannamaker, L. W.; Brink, W. R.; Rammelkamp, C. H., Jr.; and Custer, E. A.: Prevention of rheumatic fever: Treatment of the preceding streptococcal infection. J.A.M.A. 143:151, 1950.

Diamond, E. F.: Hereditary and environmental factors in the pathogenesis of rheumatic fever. Pediatrics 19:908, 1957.

Diamond, E. F.: Is there a rheumatic constitution? J. Pediat. 54:341, 1959.

Diamond, E. F. and Tentler, R.: The electroencephalogram in rheumatic fever. J.A.M.A. 182:685, 1962.

Dick, L. S. and Grant, M. D.: The nurse's role in rehabilitation of the child with rheumatic fever. Public Health Rep. 79:533, 1964.

Diehl, A. M.; Hamilton, T. R.; Keeling, I. C.; and May, J. S.: Long-acting repository penicillin in prophylaxis of recurrent rheumatic fever. J.A.M.A. 155:1466, 1954.

Dixon, A. St. J. and Bywaters, E. G. L.: Methods of assessing therapy in chorea with special reference to the use of A.C.T.H. Arch. Dis. Child. 27:161, 1952.

Dodge, K. G.; Baldwin, J. S.; and Weber, M. W.: The prophylactic use of sulfanilamide in children with inactive rheumatic fever. J. Pediat. 24:483, 1944.

Done, A. K.; Ely, R. S.; Ainger, L. E.; Seely, J. R.; and Kelley, V. C.: Therapy of acute rheumatic fever. Pediatrics 15:522, 1955.

Dorfman, A.; Gross, J. I.; and Lorinez, A. E.: The treatment of acute rheumatic fever. Pediatrics 27:692, 1961.

Eastman, N. J.: In: Williams Obstetrics, page 781. Appleton-Century-Crofts, Inc., New York, 1956.

Edwards, J. E. and Burchell, H. B.: Pathologic anatomy of mitral insufficiency. Proc. Mayo Clin. 33:497, 1958.

Elling, R.; Whittemore, R.; and Green, M.: Patient participation in a pediatric program. J. Health Hum. Behav. 1:183, 1960.

Elliott, S. D.: Bacteriaemia following tonsillectomy. Lancet 2:589, 1939.

Ellis, L. B.: Recurrent mitral stenosis. Mod. Conc. Cardiov. Dis. 33:851, 1964.

Elster, S. K.; Braunwald, E.; and Wood, H. F.: A study of C-reactive protein in the serum of patients with congestive heart failure. Amer. Heart J. 51:533, 1956.

Elster, S. K. and Wood, H. F.: Studies of C-reactive protein in patients with rheumatic heart disease. 1. Lack of correlation between C-reactive protein and Aschoff bodies in left auricular appendage biopsies. Amer. Heart J. 50:706, 1955.

Epidemiology Unit Number 22: Sulfadiazine resistant strains of beta hemolytic streptococci: Appearance during the course of sulfadiazine prophylaxis at a large naval training center. J.A.M.A. 129:921, 1945.

Evans, A. S. and Dick, E. C.: Acute pharyngitis and tonsillitis in University of Wisconsin students. J.A.M.A. 190:699, 1964.

Evans, J. A. P.: Discussion on management of rheumatic fever and its early complications; oral penicillin in prophylaxis of streptococcal infection and rheumatic relapse. Proc. Roy. Soc. Med. 43:206, 1950.

Feinstein, A. R. and Arevalo, A. C.: Manifestations and treatment of congestive heart failure in young patients with rheumatic heart disease. Pediatrics 33:661, 1964.

Feinstein, A. R. and DiMassa, R.: Prognostic significance of valvular involvement in acute rheumatic fever. New Eng. J. Med. 260:1001, 1959.

Feinstein, A. R. and DiMassa, R.: The unheard diastolic murmur in acute rheumatic fever. New Eng. J. Med. 260:1331, 1959.

Feinstein, A. R. and Spagnuolo, M.: Mimetic features of rheumatic-fever recurrences. New Eng. J. Med. 262:533, 1960.

Feinstein, A. R. and Spagnuolo, M.: The duration of activity in acute rheumatic fever. J.A.M.A. *175*:1117, 1961.

Feinstein, A. R. and Spagnuolo, M.: The clinical patterns of acute rheumatic fever: A reappraisal. Medicine (Balt.) *41*:279, 1962.

Feinstein, A. R.; Spagnuolo, M.; and Gill, F. A.: The rebound phenomenon in acute rheumatic fever. I. Incidence and significance. Yale J. Biol. Med. *33*:259, 1961.

Feinstein, A. R.; Spagnuolo, M.; Jonas, S.; Tursky, E.; Stern, E. K.; and Levitt, M.: Antirheumatic prophylaxis monthly with long acting injections of penicillin versus intermittent oral therapy. Circulation *30*:(Suppl. 3) 75, 1964 (Abs.).

Feinstein, A. R.; Taranta, A.; and DiMassa, R.: Errors in the diagnosis of acute rheumatic fever. New York J. Med. *60*:2835, 1960.

Feinstein, A. R.; Taube, H.; Cavalieri, R.; Schultz, S. C.; and Kryle, L.: Physical activities and rheumatic heart disease in asymptomatic patients. J.A.M.A. *180*: 1028, 1962.

Feinstein, A. R.; Wood, H. F.; Spagnuolo, M.; Taranta, A.; Jones, S.; Kleinberg, E.; and Tursky, E.: Rheumatic fever in children and adolescents. VII. Cardiac changes and sequelae. Ann. Intern. Med. *60*:(Suppl. 5) 87, 1964.

Feinstein, A. R.; Wood, H. F.; Spagnuolo, M.; Taranta, A.; Tursky, E.; and Kleinberg, E.: Oral prophylaxis of recurrent rheumatic fever. Sulfadiazine vs. a double daily dose of penicillin. J.A.M.A. *188*:489, 1964.

Feldt, R. H.: Sulfanilamide as a prophylactic measure in recurrent rheumatic infection: Controlled study involving 131 "patient-seasons." Amer. J. Med. Sci. *207*:483, 1944.

Fenn, G. K.; Kerr, W. J.; Levy, R. L.; Strand, W. D.; and White, P. D.: Reexamination of 4,994 men rejected for general military service because of diagnosis of cardiovascular defects. Amer. Heart J. *27*:435, 1944.

Ferencz, C.; Markowitz, M.; and Bunim, J. J.: The effect of large doses of prednisone on acute rheumatic fever. Observations on the treatment of seventeen patients with carditis with a two year follow-up. Amer. J. Dis. Child. *97*:561, 1959.

Fischel, E. E.; Frank, C. W.; Boltax, A. J.; and Arcasoy, M.: Observations on the treatment of rheumatic fever with salicylate, ACTH, and cortisone. II. Combined salicylate and corticoid therapy and attempts at rebound suppression. Arthritis Rheum. *1*:351, 1958.

Fletcher, T. F.: Sydenham's chorea treated with cortisone. Penn. Med. J. *63*:63, 1960.

Fogel, D. H.: The innocent (functional) cardiac murmur in children. Pediatrics *19*:793, 1957.

Fogel, D. H.: The innocent systolic murmur in children: A clinical study of its incidence and characteristics. Amer. Heart J. *59*:844, 1960.

Foster, F. P.; McEachern, G. C.; Miller, J. H.; Ball, F. E.; Higley, C. S.; and Warren, H. A.: The treatment of acute rheumatic fever with penicillin. J.A.M.A. *126*: 281, 1944.

Frahm, C. J.; Braunwald, E.; and Morrow, A. G.: Congenital aortic regurgitation. Clinical and hemodynamic findings in four patients. Amer. J. Med. *31*:63, 1961.

Frank, P. F. and Miller, L. F.: Antagonistic effect of a penicillinase-producing staphylococcus on penicillin therapy of a streptococcal throat infection. Amer. J. Med. Sci. *243*:582, 1962.

Freeman, V. J.: Studies on the virulence of bacteriophage-infected strains of Corynebacterium diphtheriae. J. Bact. *61*:675, 1951.

Freimer, E. H.; Krause, R. M.; and McCarty, M.: Studies of L forms and protoplasts of group A streptococci. I. Isolation, growth and bacteriologic characteristics. J. Exp. Med. *110*:853, 1959.

Friedman, S.; Ash, R.; Harris, T. N.; and Lee, H. F.: Acute benign pericarditis in childhood: Comparisons with rheumatic pericarditis, and therapeutic effects of ACTH and cortisone. Pediatrics 9:551, 1952.

Friedman, S.; Harris, T. N.; and Caddell, J. L.: Long-term effects of ACTH and cortisone therapy in rheumatic fever. J. Pediat. *60*:55, 1962.

Friedman, S.; Robie, W. A.; and Harris, T. N.: Occurrence of innocent adventitious cardiac sounds in childhood. Pediatrics 4:782, 1949.

Friedman, S. and Wells, C. R. E.: Experience in secondary screening of cardiac suspects of school age. J. Pediat. *49*:410, 1956.

Galdston, I.: The rheumatic child and his world: An ecologic speculation. Pediatrics 19:916, 1957.

Gale, A. H.; Gillespie, W. A.; and Perry, C. B.: Oral penicillin in the prophylaxis of streptococcal infection in rheumatic children. Lancet 2:61, 1952.

Gardiner, J. H. and Keith, J. D.: Prevalence of heart disease in Toronto children. Pediatrics 7:713, 1951.

Garrod, L. P. and Waterworth, P. M.: The risks of dental extraction during penicillin treatment. Brit. Heart J. 24:39, 1962.

Gavrin, J. B.; Tursky, E.; Albam, B.; and Feinstein, A. R.: Rheumatic fever in children and adolescents. A long-term epidemiologic study of subsequent prophylaxis, streptococcal infections and clinical sequelae. II. Maintenance and preservation of the population. Ann. Intern. Med. 60: (Suppl. 5) 18, 1964.

Gerstley, J. R.; Wile, S. A.; Falstein, E. I.; and Gayle, M.: Chorea: Is it a manifestation of rheumatic fever? J. Pediat. 6:42, 1935.

Gelli, G.: Recent experience in the treatment of rheumatic carditis with hormones and salicylate. Ann. Rheum. Dis. 14:306, 1955.

Gibson, M. L. and Fisher, G. R.: Early ambulation in rheumatic fever. A.M.A. J. Dis. Child. 96:575, 1958 (Abst.).

Gibson, S.: Auricular fibrillation in childhood and adolescence. J.A.M.A. 117:96, 1941.

Gilbert-Queralto, J.; Paravisini-Paria, J.; Torner-Soler, M.; and Gauisi-Gene, C.: Mitral commissurotomy in younger age groups. Fourth World Congress of Cardiology, Mexico City, October, 1962, Abstracts, p. 142.

Giles, C. and Shuttleworth, E. M.: Post-mortem findings in 46 influenza deaths. Lancet 2:1224, 1957.

Gitlin, D.; Craig, J. M.; and Janeway, J. A.: Studies on the nature of fibrinoid in the collagen diseases. Amer. J. Path. 33:55, 1957.

Glaser, G. H. and Merritt, H. H.: Effects of corticotropin (ACTH) and cortisone on disorders of the nervous system. J.A.M.A. 148:898, 1952.

Glaser, H. H.; Lynn, D. B.; Harrison, G. S.: Comprehensive medical care for handicapped children. I. Patterns of anxiety in mothers of children with rheumatic fever. Amer. J. Dis. Child. 102:344, 1961.

Glover, J. A.: Milroy lectures on the incidence of rheumatic diseases. I. The incidence of acute rheumatism. Lancet 1:499, 1930.

Glynn, A. A.; Glynn, L. E.; and Halborow, E. J.: Secretion of blood-group substances in rheumatic fever. Brit. Med. J. 2:266, 1959.

Glynn, L. E. and Halborow, E. J.: Relation between blood groups. Secretion status and susceptibility to rheumatic fever. Arthritis Rheum. 4:203, 1961.

Goerner, J. R.; Massell, B. F.; and Jones, T. D.: Use of penicillin in the treatment of carriers of beta-hemolytic streptococci among patients with rheumatic fever. New Eng. J. Med. 237:576, 1947.

Gold, H. and DeGraff, A. C.: Studies on digitalis in ambulatory cardiac patients; digitalization by small dose method; use of digitalis in children. J.A.M.A. 92:1421, 1929.

Goldring, D.; Behrer, M. R.; Brown, G.; and Elliot, G.: Rheumatic pneumonitis. Part II. Report on the clinical and laboratory findings in twenty-three patients. J. Pediat. 53:547, 1958.

Good, R. A. and Gabrielson, A. E.: Agammaglobulinemia and hypogammaglobulinemia; Relationship to the mesenchymal diseases. In: The Streptococcus, Rheumatic Fever and Glomerulonephritis, page 368. Ed. Uhr, J. W. Williams and Wilkins Co., Baltimore, 1964.

Goslings, W. R. O.; Valkenburg, H. A.; Bots, A. W.; and Lorrier, J. C.: Attack rates of streptococcal pharyngitis, rheumatic fever and glomerulonephritis in the general population. I. A controlled pilot study of streptococcal pharyngitis in one village. New Eng. J. Med. 268:687, 1963.

Grave, P. E.: Social and environmental factors in the aetiology of rheumatic fever. Med. J. Aust. 44:602, 1957.

Gray, F. G.; Quinn, R. W.; and Quinn, J. P.: A long-term survey of rheumatic and non-rheumatic families with particular reference to environment and heredity. Amer. J. Med. 13:400, 1952.

Gray, I. R.: Mitral valvotomy in the young. Lancet 2:1263, 1958.

Green, C. A.: Researches into the aetiology of acute rheumatism; rheumatic carditis; post-mortem investigation of nine consecutive cases. Ann. Rheum. Dis. *1*:86, 1939.

Greenman, L.; Weigand, F. A.; and Danowski, T. S.: Cortisone therapy in initial attacks of rheumatic carditis. Ann. Rheum. Dis. *12*:342, 1953.

Grossman, B. J. and Athreya, B.: Sources of errors in diagnosis of acute rheumatic fever in children. J.A.M.A. *182*:830, 1962.

Grossman, B. J. and Stamler, J.: Potential preventability in first attacks of acute rheumatic fever in children. J.A.M.A. *183*:985, 1963.

Guasch, J.; Vignau, A.; Mortimer, E. A.; and Rammelkamp, C. H., Jr.: Studies of the role of continuing or recurrent streptococcal infection in rheumatic valvular heart disease. Amer. J. Med. Sci. *244*:290, 1962.

Haas, R. C.; Taranta, A.; and Wood, H. F.: Effect of intramuscular injections of benzathine penicillin G on some acute-phase reactants. New Eng. J. Med. *256*:152, 1957.

Haddox, C. H. and Saslaw, M. S.: Urinary 5-methoxytryptamine in patients with rheumatic fever. J. Clin. Invest. *42*:435, 1963.

Hahan, E. O.; Houser, H. B.; Rammelkamp, C. H.; Denny, F. W.; and Wannamaker, L. W.: Effect of cortisone on acute streptococcal infections and poststreptococcal complications. J. Clin. Invest. *30*:274, 1951.

Haig-Brown, C.: Tonsillitis in Adolescents. Bailliere, Tendoll and Cox, London, 1886.

Hallidie-Smith, K. A. and Bywaters, E. G. L.: The differential diagnosis of rheumatic fever. Arch. Dis. Child. *33*:350, 1958.

Halsey, R. H.: Heart disease in children of school age. J.A.M.A. *77*:672, 1921.

Hamburger, M., Jr.; Green, M. J.; and Hamburger, V. G.: The problem of the "dangerous carrier" of hemolytic streptococci. II. Spread of infection by individuals with strongly positive nose cultures who expelled large numbers of hemolytic streptococci. J. Infect. Dis. *77*:96, 1945.

Hamlin, R. H.: Voluntary Health and Welfare Agencies in the United States. An Exploratory Study of an Ad Hoc Citizens Committee. The Schoolmasters' Press, New York, 1961.

Hansen, A. E.; Platou, R. V.; and Dwan, P. F.: Prolonged use of a sulfonamide compound in prevention of rheumatic recrudescences in children. An evaluation based on a 4 year study on 64 children. A.M.A. Amer. J. Dis. Child. *64*:963, 1942.

Harris, S. and Harris, T. N.: Serologic response to streptococcal hemolysin and hyaluronidase in streptococcal and rheumatic infection. J. Clin. Invest. *29*:351, 1950.

Harris, T. N.: The erythrocyte sedimentation rate in rheumatic fever. Its significance in adolescent and overweight children. Amer. J. Med. Sci. *210*:173, 1945.

Harris, T. N.; Friedman, S.; Needleman, H. L.; and Saltzman, H. A.: Therapeutic effects of ACTH and cortisone in rheumatic fever: Cardiologic observations in a controlled series of 100 cases. Pediatrics *17*:11, 1956.

Harvey, W. P. and Capone, M. A.: Bacterial endocarditis related to cleaning and filling of teeth: With particular reference to the inadequacy of present day knowledge and practice of antibiotic prophylaxis for all dental procedures. Amer. J. Cardiol. *7*:793, 1961.

Hawn, C. VanZ. and Janeway, C. A.: Histological and serological sequences in experimental hypersensitivity. J. Exp. Med. *85*:571, 1947.

Hayashi, J. A. and Walsh, G.: Studies of streptococcal cell walls. VI. Effects of adjuvants on the production of type-specific antibodies to cell walls and isolated M protein. J. Bact. *82*:736, 1961.

Hedley, O. F.: Rheumatic heart disease in Philadelphia hospitals. Public Health Rep. *55*:1647, 1940.

Heinzelmann, F.: Factors influencing prophylaxis behavior with respect to rheumatic fever: An exploratory study. J. Health Hum. Behav. *3*:73, 1962.

Hench, P. S.; Slocumb, C. H.; Barnes, A. R.; Smith, H. L.; Polley, H. F.; and Kendall, E. C.: Effects of adrenal cortical hormone 17-hydroxy-11-dehydrocorticosterone (Compound E) on acute phase of rheumatic fever: Preliminary report. Proc. Mayo Clin. *24*:277, 1949.

Hers, J. F. and Mulder, J.: Broad aspects of the pathology and pathogenesis of human influenza. Amer. Rev. Resp. Dis. 83(2)Pt. 2:84, 1961.

Hess, E. V.; Fink, C. W.; Taranta, A.; and Ziff, M.: Heart muscle antibodies in rheumatic fever and other diseases. J. Clin. Invest. 43:886, 1964.

Hirschhorn, K.; Schreibman, R. R.; Verbo, S.; and Gruskin, R. H.: The action of streptolysin S on peripheral lymphocytes of normal subjects and patients with acute rheumatic fever. Proc. Nat. Acad. Sci. U.S.A. 52:1151, 1964.

Hodes, R.; Gribetz, I.; and Hodes, H. L.: Abnormal occurrence of the ulnar nerve-hypothenar, muscle H-reflex in Sydenham's chorea. Pediatrics 30:49, 1962.

Holbrook, W. P.: The Army Air Forces rheumatic fever control program. J.A.M.A. 126:84, 1944.

Holmes, M. C. and Williams, R. E.: Streptococcal infections among children in a residential home. III. Some factors influencing susceptibility to infection. J. Hyg. 56:197, 1958.

Hook, E. W. and Kaye, D.: Prophylaxis of bacterial endocarditis. J. Chronic Dis. 15:635, 1962.

Houser, H. B.; Eckhardt, G. C.; Hahn, E. O.; Denny, F. W.; Wannamaker, L. W.; and Rammelkamp, C. H., Jr.: Effect of aureomycin treatment of streptococcal sore throat on the streptococcal carrier state, the immunologic response of the host and the incidence of acute rheumatic fever. Pediatrics 12:593, 1953.

Hubbard, J. P. and McKee, M. H.: The anemia of rheumatic fever. J. Pediat. 14:66, 1939.

Humphries, J. O'N. and McKusick, V. A.: The differentiation of organic and "innocent" systolic murmurs. Progr. Cardiov. Dis. 5:152, 1962.

Husson, G. S.; Blackman, M. S.; Riemenschneider, P.; and Berne, A. S.: Isolated congenital mitral insufficiency. J. Pediat. 64:248, 1964.

Illingworth, R. S.; Burke, J.; Doxiadis, S. A.; Lorber, J.; Philpott, M. G.; and Stone, D. G. H.: Salicylates in rheumatic fever; an attempt to assess their value. Quart. J. Med. 23:177, 1954.

Illingworth, R. S.; Lorber, J.; Holt, K. S.; Rendle-Short, J.; Jowett, G. H.; and Gibson, W. M.: Acute rheumatic fever in children. A comparison of six forms of treatment in 200 cases. Lancet 2:653, 1957.

Jager, B. V. and Alway, R.: The treatment of acute rheumatic fever with large doses of sodium salicylate with special reference to dose management and toxic manifestations. Amer. J. Med. Sci. 211:273, 1946.

James, W. E. S.; Badger, G. F.; and Dingle, J. H.: A study of illness in a group of Cleveland families. XIX. The epidemiology of the acquisition of group A streptococci and of associated illnesses. New Eng. J. Med. 262:687, 1960.

Jhaveri, S.; Czoniczer, G.; Reider, R. B.; and Massell, B. F.: Relatively benign "pure" mitral regurgitation of rheumatic origin. Circulation 22:39, 1960.

Johnson, E. E.; Stollerman, G. H.; and Grossman, B. J.: Rheumatic recurrences in patients not receiving continuous prophylaxis. J.A.M.A. 190:407, 1964.

Johnson, R. D. and Hartman, T. L.: Sulfadiazine resistant streptococcal infections in a civilian community. J. Clin. Invest. 26:325, 1947.

Jones criteria (modified) for guidance in the diagnosis of rheumatic fever. Mod. Conc. Cardiov. Dis. 24:291, 1955.

Jones, T. D.: The diagnosis of rheumatic fever. J.A.M.A. 126:481, 1944.

Jones, T. D. and Bland, E. F.: Clinical significance of chorea as a manifestation of rheumatic fever; a study in prognosis. J.A.M.A. 105:571, 1935.

Jones, T. D. and Bland, E. F.: Rheumatic fever and heart disease; completed 10-year observations on 1000 patients. Trans. Ass. Amer. Physicians 57:265, 1942.

Kagan, B. M. and Mirman, B.: Sydenham's chorea, a syndrome for differential diagnosis. J. Pediat. 31:322, 1947.

Kagan, G. J.: L forms of B-hemolytic streptococcus and their pathogenic role. International (8) Congress for Microbiology, Abstracts, p. 125, 1962.

Kaplan, M. H.: Immunologic relation of streptococcal and tissue antigens. I. Properties of an antigen in certain strains of group A streptococci exhibiting an immuologic cross-reaction with human heart tissue. J. Immun. 90:595, 1963.

Kaplan, M. H.; Meyeserian, M.; and Kushner, I.: Immunologic studies of heart tissue. IV. Serologic reactions with human heart tissue as revealed by immunofluorescent methods: Isoimmune, Wasserman and autoimmune reactions. J. Exp. Med. 113:17, 1961.

Kay, E. B. and Zimmerman, H. A.: Surgical treatment of mitral stenosis: Open versus closed technics. Amer. J. Cardiol. 10:1, 1962.

Keil, H.: Rheumatic erythemas; A critical survey. Ann. Intern. Med. 11:2223, 1938.

Keith, J. D.: Overstimulation of the vagus nerve in rheumatic fever. Quart. J. Med. 7:29, 1938.

Keith, J. D.: Congenital mitral insufficiency. Progr. Cardiov. Dis. 5:264, 1962.

Keith, J. D. and Ross, A.: Observations on salicylate therapy in rheumatic fever. Canad. Med. Ass. J. 52:554, 1945.

Kelley, V. C.: Rationale for hormone therapy in rheumatic fever. Ann. N. Y. Acad. Sci. 61:369, 1955.

Kelley, V. C. and Ely, R. S.: Production and metabolism of adrenocorticosteroids in connective tissue disease. Ann. N. Y. Acad. Sci. 86:1115, 1960.

Kelley, V. C.; Good, R. A.; and McQuarrie, I.: Serum mucoproteins in children in health and disease with special reference to rheumatic fever. Pediatrics 5:824, 1950.

Kellner, A.; Freeman, E. B.; and Carlson, A. S.: Neutralizing antibodies to streptococcal diphosphopyridine nucleotidase in the serum of experimental animals and human beings. J. Exper. Med. 108:299, 1958.

Kernohan, J. W.; Woltman, H. W.; and Barnes, A. R.: Involvement of the nervous system associated with endocarditis. Neuropsychiatric and neuropathologic observations in 42 cases of fatal outcome. Arch. Neurol. Psychiat. 42:789, 1939.

Kerr, A., Jr.: Subacute Bacterial Endocarditis. Charles C Thomas, Springfield, Ill., 1955.

Kerr, A., Jr.: Bacterial endocarditis—revisited. Mod. Conc. Cardiov. Dis. 33:831, 1964.

Kilbourne, E. D. and Loge, J. P.: The comparative effects of continuous and intermittent penicillin therapy on the formation of antistreptolysin in hemolytic streptococcal pharyngitis. J. Clin. Invest. 27:418, 1948.

Kjems, E.: Studies on streptococcal bacteriophages. I. Technique of isolating phage-producing strains. Acta path. Microbiol. Scand. 36:433, 1955.

Kjems, E.: Studies on streptococcal bacteriophages. 4. The occurrence of lysogenic strains among group A haemolytic streptococci. Acta path. Microbiol. Scand. 49:199, 1960.

Klinge, F.: Der Rheumatismus. J. F. Bergmoun, Munich, 1933.

Kohn, K. H.; Milzer, A.; and MacLean, H.: Oral penicillin prophylaxis of recurrences of rheumatic fever. Interim report after a three year study. J.A.M.A. 142:20, 1950.

Krause, R. M.: Studies on bacteriophages of hemolytic streptococci. I. Factors influencing the interaction of phage and susceptible host cell. J. Exp. Med. 106:365, 1957.

Krause, R. M. and McCarty, M.: Studies on the chemical structure of the streptococcal cell wall. I. The identification of a mucopeptide in the cell walls of groups A and A-variant streptococci. J. Exp. Med. 114:127, 1961.

Krause, R. M. and Rammelkamp, C. H., Jr.: Studies of the carrier state following infection with group A streptococci. II. Infectivity of streptococci isolated during acute pharyngitis and during the carrier state. J. Clin. Invest. 41:575, 1962.

Krause, R. M.; Rammelkamp, C. H., Jr.; Denny, F. W., Jr.; and Wannamaker, L. W.: Studies of the carrier state following infection with group A streptococci. I. Effect of climate. J. Clin. Invest. 41:568, 1962.

Kroop, I. G.; Heffer, E. T.; and Shackman, N. H.: An evaluation of electrophoresis in rheumatic fever. Amer. Heart J. 48:612, 1954.

Krumwiede, E. and Kuttner, A. G.: Growth inhibitory substance for influenza group of organisms in blood of various animal species: Use of blood of various animals as selective media for detection of hemolytic streptococci in throat cultures. J. Exper. Med. 67:429, 1938.

Kuharic, H. A.; Roberts, C. E.; and Kirby, W. M. M.: Tetracycline resistance of group A beta hemolytic streptococci. J.A.M.A. 174:1779, 1960.

Kuhns, W. J. and McCarty, M.: Studies of diphtheria antitoxin in rheumatic fever subjects: Analysis of reactions to the Schick test and of antitoxin responses following hyperimmunization with diphtheria toxoid. J. Clin. Invest. 33:759, 1954.

Kundsin, R. B. and Miller, J. M.: Significance of the staphylococcus aureus carrier state in the treatment of disease due to group A streptococci. New Eng. J. Med. 271:1395, 1964.

Kuschner, M. and Levieff, L.: Correlation between active rheumatic lesions in the left auricular appendage and elsewhere in the heart. Amer. J. Med. Sci. 226:290, 1953.

Kuttner, A. G. and Krumwiede, E.: Observations on the effect of streptococcal upper respiratory infections on rheumatic children: A three-year study. J. Clin. Invest. 20:273, 1941.

Kuttner, A. G. and Krumwiede, E.: Observations on the epidemiology of streptococcal pharyngitis and the relation of streptococcal carriers to the occurrence of outbreaks. J. Clin. Invest. 23:139, 1944.

Kuttner, A. G. and Lenert, T. F.: The occurrence of bacteriostatic properties in the blood of patients after recovery from streptococcal pharyngitis. J. Clin. Invest. 23:151, 1944.

Kuttner, A. G. and Mayer, F. E.: Carditis during second attacks of rheumatic fever. New Eng. J. Med. 268:1259, 1963.

Kuttner, A. G. and Reyersbach, G.: The value of special radiologic procedures in detecting cardiac enlargement in children with rheumatic heart disease. Amer. Heart J. 18:213, 1939.

Kuttner, A. G. and Reyersbach, G.: The prevention of streptococcal upper respiratory infections and rheumatic recurrences in rheumatic children by the prophylactic use of sulfanilamide. J. Clin. Invest. 22:77, 1943.

Lancefield, R. C.: Specific relationship of cell composition to biological activity of hemolytic streptococci. Harvey Lect. 36:251, 1940-1941.

Lancefield, R. C.: Cellular constituents of group A streptococci concerned in antigenicity and virulence. In: Streptococcal Infections, page 3. Ed. McCarty, M. Columbia University Press, New York, 1954.

Lancefield, R. C.: Current knowledge of type-specific M antigens of group A streptococci. J. Immun. 89:307, 1962.

Lannigan, R.: The rheumatic process in the left auricular appendage. J. Path. Bact. 77:49, 1959.

Lannigan, R. and Zaki, S.: Electron microscopic appearances of rheumatic lesions in the left auricular appendage in mitral stenosis. Nature 198:898, 1963.

Lattimer, A.; Siegel, A. C.; and DeCelles, J.: Comparison of the recovery of beta hemolytic streptococci by direct plating and mail-in methods. Amer. J. Public Health 53:1594, 1963.

Lees, D. B.: The treatment of some acute visceral inflammations; acute rheumatic carditis and pericarditis. Brit. Med. J. 2:1318, 1903.

Lendrum, B. L.; Simon, A. J.; and Mack, I.: Relation of duration of bed rest in acute rheumatic fever to heart disease present 2 to 14 years later. Pediatrics 24:389, 1959.

Lessof, M. and Brigden, W.: Systolic murmurs in healthy children and in children with rheumatic fever. Lancet 2:673, 1957.

Levander-Lindgren, M.: Electrocardiographic studies in scarlet fever. Acta Paediat. (Stockholm) Suppl. 91:1, 1952.

Levine, S. A. and Harvey, W. P.: Clinical Auscultation of the Heart. 2nd Ed. W. B. Saunders Co., Philadelphia, 1959.

Levy, M. J. and Edwards, J. E.: Anatomy of mitral insufficiency. Progr. Cardiov. Dis. 5:119, 1962.

Lewis-Jonsson, J.: Chorea: Its nomenclature, etiology and epidemiology in a clinical material from Malmohus County. 1910-1944. Acta Paediat. (Stockholm) Suppl. 76:1, 1949.

Lietman, P. S. and Bywaters, E. G. L.: Pericarditis in juvenile rheumatoid arthritis. Pediatrics 32:855, 1963.

Lim, W. N. and Wilson, M. G.: Comparison of the recurrence rate of rheumatic carditis among children receiving penicillin by mouth prophylactically or on indication. New Eng. J. Med. 262:321, 1960.

Luisada, A. A.; Haring, O. M.; and Zilli, A. B.: Apical diastolic murmurs simulating mitral stenosis: graphic differentiation. Ann. Intern. Med. *42*:644, 1955.

Lurie, P. R. and Shumacker, H. B., Jr.: Mitral commissurotomy in childhood. Pediatrics *13*:454, 1954.

McCarty, M.: The occurrence of nucleases in culture filtrates of group A hemolytic streptococci. J. Exp. Med. *88*:181, 1948.

McCarty, M. (Ed.): Streptococcal Infections. Columbia University Press, New York, 1954.

McCarty, M.: Nature of rheumatic fever. Circulation *14*:1138, 1956.

McCarty, M.: The streptococcal cell wall and its biologic significance. *In*: The Streptococcus, Rheumatic Fever and Glomerulonephritis, p. 3. Ed. Uhr, J. W. Williams and Wilkins Co., Baltimore, 1964.

McCarty, M.: *In*: The Streptococcus, Rheumatic Fever and Glomerulonephritis, page 204. Ed. Uhr, J. W. Williams and Wilkins Co., Baltimore, 1964.

McFarland, R. B.: Reactions to benzathine penicillin. New Eng. J. Med. *259*:62, 1958.

McKusick, V. A.: Cardiovascular Sound in Health and Disease. Williams and Wilkins Co., Baltimore, 1958.

Maclagan, T.: The treatment of acute rheumatism by Salicin. Lancet *1*:342, 1876.

MacLeod, C. M.: Hypersensitivity and disease. *In*: Cellular and Humoral Aspects of the Hypersensitivity States, page 615. Ed. Lawrence, H. S. Hoeber-Harper, New York, 1959.

Madsen, T. and Kalbak, K.: Investigations on rheumatic fever subsequent to some epidemics of septic sore throat (especially milk epidemics). Acta path. Microbiol. Scand. *17*:305, 1940.

Magarey, F. R.: Pathogenesis of mitral stenosis. Brit. Med. J. *1*:856, 1951.

Maliner, M. M. and Amsterdam, S. D.: Oral penicillin in the prophylaxis of recurrent rheumatic fever. J. Pediat. *31*:658, 1947.

Maliner, M. M.; Amsterdam, S. D.; and Arreche, C. C.: Further studies on oral penicillin in the prophylaxis of recurrent rheumatic fever. J. Pediat. *35*:145, 1949.

Mallen, M. S. and Castillo, F.: Estudios Sabre la Genética del Rheumatismo Cardioarticular. I. La Hipótesis de un Gene Recésivo. Arch. Inst. Cardiol. Mex. *22*: 136, 1952.

Manchester, R. C.: Rheumatic fever in naval enlisted personnel. II. Effectiveness of intensive salicylate therapy in cases of acute infection. Arch. Intern. Med. *78*:170, 1946.

Marienfeld, C. J.; Robins, M.; Sandidge, R. P.; and Findlan, C.: Rheumatic fever and rheumatic heart disease among U.S. college freshmen, 1956-60. Prevalence, prophylaxis. Public Health Rep. *79*:789, 1964.

Markowitz, M.: Observations on an epidemic of streptococcal infections and recurrences of rheumatic fever among children treated with penicillin. Pediatrics *20*:257, 1957 B.

Markowitz, M.: Analysis of diagnostic errors in rheumatic fever and rheumatic heart disease. (unpublished observations) 1960.

Markowitz, M.: Cultures of the respiratory tract in pediatric practice. Amer. J. Dis. Child. *105*:12, 1963 A.

Markowitz, M.: Studies on type-specific streptococcal antibodies as indicators of previous streptococcal infections in rheumatic and non-rheumatic children. J. Clin. Invest. *42*:409, 1963 B.

Markowitz, M.; Bruton, H. D.; Kuttner, A. G.; and Cluff, L. E.: The bacteriologic findings, streptococcal immune response and renal complications in children with impetigo. Pediatrics (in press) 1965.

Markowitz, M.; Ferencz, C.; and Bonet, A.: A comparison of oral and intramuscular benzathine penicillin G for the prevention of streptococcal infections and recurrences of rheumatic fever. Pediatrics *19*:201, 1957 A.

Markowitz, M. and Hemphill, W.: A comparison of oral benzathine penicillin G and sulfonamides for the prevention of streptococcal infections and recurrences of rheumatic fever. Pediatrics *15*:509, 1955.

Markowitz, M. and Kuttner, A. G.: A study of the absorption and excretion of oral penicillin in children. J. Pediat. *31*:195, 1947.

Markowitz, M. and Kuttner, A. G.: The effect of intensive and prolonged therapy with cortisone and hydrocortisone in first attacks of rheumatic carditis. Pediatrics 16:325, 1955.

Marshall, H. W.; Woodward, E., Jr.; and Wood, E. H.: Hemodynamic methods for differentiation of mitral stenosis and regurgitation. Amer. J. Cardiol. 2:24, 1958.

Massell, B. F.: The diagnosis and treatment of rheumatic fever and rheumatic carditis. Med. Clin. N. Amer. 42:1343, 1958.

Massell, B. F.; Amezcua, F.; and Pelargonio, S.: Evolving picture of rheumatic fever. Data from 40 years at the House of the Good Samaritan. J.A.M.A. 188:287, 1964.

Massell, B. F.; Dow, J. W.; and Jones, T. D.: Orally administered penicillin in patients with rheumatic fever, J.A.M.A. 138:1030, 1948.

Massell, B. F.; Fyler, D. C.; and Roy, S. B.: The clinical picture of rheumatic fever. Diagnosis, immediate prognosis, course and therapeutic implications. Amer. J. Cardiol. 1:436, 1958.

Massell, B. F.; Jhaveri, S.; and Czoniczer, G.: Therapy and other factors influencing the course of rheumatic heart disease. Circulation 20:737, 1959.

Massell, B. F.; Jhaveri, S.; Czoniczer, G.; and Barnet, R.: Treatment of rheumatic fever and rheumatic carditis. Observations providing a basis for the selection of aspirin or adrenocortical steroids. Med. Clin. N. Amer. 45:1349, 1961.

Massell, B. F. and Jones, T. D.: The effect of sulfanilamide on rheumatic fever and chorea. New Eng. J. Med. 218:876, 1938.

Massell, B. F.; Sturgis, G. P.; Knobloch, J. D.; Hall, T. N.; and Norcross, P.: Prevention of rheumatic fever by prompt penicillin therapy of hemolytic streptococcic respiratory infections. J.A.M.A. 146:1469, 1951.

Massie, R. W. and Stahlman, M.: Serum oxaloacetic transaminase activity in acute rheumatic fever. A.M.A. J. Dis. Child. 95:469, 1958.

Mathy, W. E.: Rheumatic fever survey, 1958. Heart Disease Control Program, Minnesota Department of Health.

Mattison, B. F.; Lambert, E. C.; and Mosher, W. E.: Cardiac screening in a school health program. New York J. Med. 53:2966, 1953.

Mauer, A. M.: The early anemia of acute rheumatic fever. Pediatrics 27:707, 1961.

Maxted, W. R.: The use of bacitracin for identifying group A haemolytic streptococci. J. Clin. Path. 6:224, 1953.

Maxted, W. R.: Streptococcal bacteriophages. In: The Streptococcus, Rheumatic Fever and Glomerulonephritis, page 25. Ed. Uhr, J. W. Williams and Wilkins Co., Baltimore, 1964.

Mayer, F. E.; Doyle, E. F.; Herrera, L.; and Brownell, K. D.: Declining severity of first attack of rheumatic fever. Amer. J. Dis. Child. 105:146, 1963.

Medearis, D. N.; Neill, C. A.; and Markowitz, M.: Influenza and cardiopulmonary disease. (I.) Mod. Conc. Cardiov. Dis. 32:809, 1963.

Medearis, D N.; Neill, C. A.; and Markowitz, M.: Influenza and cardiopulmonary disease. (II.) Mod. Conc. Cardiov. Dis. 32:813, 1963.

Meyer, R. J. and Haggerty, R. J.: Streptococcal infections in families. Factors altering individual susceptibility. Pediatrics 29:539, 1962.

Miller, J. M.; Staucer, S. L.; and Massell, B. F.: A controlled study of beta hemolytic streptococcal infection in rheumatic families. I. Streptococcal disease among healthy siblings. Amer. J. Med. 25:825, 1958.

Miller, R. A.; Smith, J.; Stamler, J.; Hahneman, B.; Paul, M. H.; Abrams, I.; Hait, G.; Edelman, J.; Willard, J.; and Stevens, W.: The detection of heart disease in children. Results of a mass field trial with use of tape-recorded heart sounds. Circulation 25:85, 1962.

Milzer, A.; Kohn, K. H.; and MacLean, H.: Oral prophylaxis of rheumatic fever with penicillin. Resistant hemolytic streptococci. J.A.M.A. 136:536, 1948.

Mirowski, M.; Rosenstein, B. J.; and Markowitz, M.: A comparison of atrioventricular conduction in normal children and in patients with rheumatic fever, glomerulonephritis, and acute febrile illnesses. A quantitative study with determination of the P-R index. Pediatrics 33:334, 1964.

Moffet, H. L.; Cramblett, G. H.; and Smith, A.: Group A streptococcal infections in a children's home. II. Clinical and epidemiologic patterns of illness. Pediatrics 33:11, 1964.

Mogabgab, W. J. and Pelon, W.: An outbreak of pharyngitis due to tetracycline-resistant group A, type 12 streptococci. A.M.A. J. Dis. Child. 96:696, 1958.

Mohler, D. N.; Wallin, D. G.; and Dreyfus, E. G.: Studies in home treatment of streptococcal disease. I. Failure of patients to take penicillin by mouth as prescribed. New Eng. J. Med. 252:1116, 1955.

Monty, C. P.: Prognosis of "observation hip" in children. Arch. Dis. Child. 37:539, 1962.

Moody, M. D.; Siegel, A. C.; Pittman, B.; and Winter, C. C.: Fluorescent-antibody identification of group A streptococci from throat swabs. Amer. J. Public Health 53:1083, 1963.

More, R. H.; Waugh, D.; and Kobernick, S. D.: Cardiac lesions produced in rabbits by massive injections of bovine serum gamma globulin. J. Exp. Med. 89:555, 1949.

Morris, A. J.; Chamovitz, R.; Catanzaro, F. J.; and Rammelkamp, C. H., Jr.: Prevention of rheumatic fever by treatment of previous streptococcic infections. Effect of sulfadiazine. J.A.M.A. 160:114, 1956.

Morris, A. J. and Rammelkamp, C. H., Jr.: Benzathine penicillin G in the prevention of streptococci infections. J.A.M.A. 165:664, 1957.

Mortimer, E. A. and Rammelkamp, C. H., Jr.: Prophylaxis of rheumatic fever. Circulation 14:1144, 1956.

Mortimer, E. A., Jr.; Vaisman, B. S.; Vigneau, I. A.; Guasch, L. J.; Schuster, C. A.; Rakita, L.; Krause, R. M.; Roberts, R.; and Rammelkamp, C. H., Jr.: The effect of penicillin on acute rheumatic fever and valvular heart disease. New Eng. J. Med. 260:101, 1959.

Morton, W.; Hoffman, M. S.; Cleeve, R. L.; and Dodge, H. J.: Comparison of three methods of screening for pediatric heart disease. J.A.M.A. 169:1169, 1959.

Murphy, G. E.: Nature of rheumatic heart disease. Medicine (Balt.) 39:289, 1960.

Mustacchi, P.; Shevins, R.; Miller, J. J.: Congenital malformations of the heart and the great vessels. J.A.M.A. 183:241, 1963.

Neimann, N.; Pierson, M.; Petit, J.; and Bouchet, J. L.: Considérations étiologiques sur la chorée de Sydenham. Pédiatrie 18:263, 1963 (Fr.).

Nixon, P. G. F.: The third heart sound in mitral regurgitation. Brit. Heart J. 23:677, 1961.

Noonan, J. A. and Spencer, F. C.: Surgical treatment of rheumatic heart disease in childhood. Circulation 30:(Suppl. 3) 133, 1964 (Abs.).

Nydick, I.; Tang, J.; Stollerman, G. H.; Wroblewski, F.; and LaDue, J. S.: The influence of rheumatic fever on serum concentrations of the enzyme, glutamic oxalacetic transaminase. Circulation 12:795, 1955.

Paradise, J. L.: Sydenham's chorea without evidence of rheumatic fever. Report of its association with the Henoch-Schönlein syndrome, and with systemic lupus erythematosus, and review of the literature. New Eng. J. Med. 263:625, 1960.

Paul, J. R.: Epidemiology of Rheumatic Fever. American Heart Association, New York, 1957.

Paul, J. R. and Leddy, P. A.: The social incidence of rheumatic heart disease. A statistical study in Yale University students. Amer. J. Med. Sci. 184:597, 1932.

Paulin, S. and Mannheimer, E.: The physiological heart murmur in children. Acta Paediat. (Stockholm) 46:438, 1957.

Perloff, J. K. and Harvey, W. P.: Auscultatory and phonocardiographic manifestations of pure mitral regurgitation. Progr. Cardiov. Dis. 5:172, 1962.

Perry, C. B.: Erythema marginatum (rheumaticum). Arch. Dis. Child. 12:233, 1937.

Perry, C. B. and Robert, J. A. F.: Study on the variability in the incidence of rheumatic heart disease within the city of Bristol. Brit. Med. J. (Suppl) 2:154, 1937.

Phibbs, B.; Becker, D.; Lowe, C. R.; Holmes, R.; Fowler, R.; Scott, O. K.; Roberts, K.; Watson, W.; and Malott, R.: The Casper Project—an enforced mass-culture streptococcic control program. I. Clinical aspects. J.A.M.A. 166:1113, 1958.

Poskanzer, D. C.; Feldman, H. A.; Beadenkopf, W. G.; Kuroda, K.; Duslane, A.; and Diamond, E. L.: Epidemiology of civilian streptococcal outbreaks before and after penicillin prophylaxis. Amer. J. Public Health 46:1513, 1956.

Potter, E. V.; Stollerman, G. H.; and Siegel, A. C.: Recall of type specific antibodies in man by injections of streptococcal cell walls. J. Clin. Invest. 41:301, 1962.

Poynton, F. J. and Holmes, G. M.: Lancet 2. Reprinted in Poynton, F. J. and Payne, A. Researches in Rheumatism. London, 1913.

Quinn, R. W.; Denny, F. W.; and Riley, H. D.: Natural occurrence of hemolytic streptococci in normal school children. Amer. J. Public Health 47:995, 1957.

Quinn, R. W.; Liao, S. J.; and Quinn, J. P.: An environmental and sociological study of rheumatic heart disease in school children from four Connecticut communities. Amer. J. Public Health 40:1285, 1950.

Rammelkamp, C. H.; Denny, F. W.; and Wannamaker, L. W.: Studies on the epidemiology of rheumatic fever in the armed services. In: Rheumatic Fever. A Symposium, page 72. Ed. Thomas, L. University of Minnesota Press, Minneapolis, 1952.

Rammelkamp, C. H., Jr. and Stolzer, B. L.: The latent period before the onset of acute rheumatic fever. Yale J. Biol. Med. 34:386, 1961.

Rammelkamp, C. H.; Wannamaker, L. W.; and Denny, F. W.: The epidemiology and prevention of rheumatic fever. Bull. N. Y. Acad. Med. 28:321, 1952.

Rantz, L. A.; Boisvert, P. J.; and Spink, W. W.: Etiology and pathogenesis of rheumatic fever. Arch. Intern. Med. 76:131, 1945.

Rantz, L. A.; Maroney, M.; and DiCaprio, J. M.: Antistreptolysin O response following hemolytic streptococcal infection in early childhood. Arch. Intern. Med. 87:360, 1951.

Rantz, L. A. and Randall, E.: A modification of the technic for determination of the antistreptolysin titer. Proc. Soc. Exp. Biol. Med. 59:22, 1945.

Rantz, L. A.; Randall, E.; and Rantz, H. H.: Antistreptolysin "O". A study of this antibody in health and in hemolytic streptococcus respiratory disease in man. Amer. J. Med. 5:3, 1948.

Rantz, L. A.; Randall, E.; and Rantz, H. H.: Immunization of human beings with group A hemolytic streptococci. Amer. J. Med. 6:424, 1949.

Rantz, L. A.; Spink, W. W.; and Boisvert, P. J.: Abnormalities in the electrocardiogram following hemolytic streptococcus sore throat. Arch. Intern. Med. 77:66, 1946.

Ravin, A. and Nice, C. M.: The angle of clearance of the left ventricle. Ann. Intern. Med. 36:1413, 1952.

Reale, A.; Colella, C.; and Bruno, A. M.: Mitral stenosis in childhood: Clinical and therapeutic aspects. Amer. Heart J. 66:15, 1963.

Reid, J.: Does sodium salicylate cure rheumatic fever? Quart. J. Med. 17:139, 1948.

Reinhold, J.: The survival of transfused red cells in acute rheumatic fever with reference to a latent haemolytic mechanism. Arch. Dis. Child. 29:201, 1954.

Reinmann, H. A.: Pneumonia. Charles C Thomas, Springfield, Ill., 1954.

Reyersbach, G. and Kuttner, A. G.: Studies on the auriculoventricular conduction time of normal children and of rheumatic children without signs of rheumatic activity. Amer. Heart J. 20:573, 1940.

Rich, A. R.: Hypersensitivity in disease with especial reference to periarteritis nodosa, rheumatic fever, disseminated lupus erythematosus and rheumatoid arthritis. Harvey Lect. 42:106, 1946-1947.

Rich, A. R. and Gregory, J. E.: On the anaphylactic nature of rheumatic pneumonitis. Bull. Johns Hopkins Hosp. 73:465, 1943.

Robey, W. H.: A cardiac survey of children in Boston public schools. Nation's Health 9:21, 1927.

Robinson, L.; Kraus, F. W.; Lazansky, J. P.; Wheeler, R. E.; Gordon, S.; and Johnson, V.: Bacteremias of dental origin. I. A review of the literature. Oral Surg. 3:519, 1950.

Robinson, L.; Kraus, F. W.; Lazansky, J. P.; Wheeler, R. E.; Gordon, S.; and Johnson, V.: Bacteremias of dental origin. II. A study of the factors influencing occurrence and detection. Oral Surg. 3:923, 1950.

Robinson, R. W.: Effect of atropine upon the prolongation of the P-R interval found in acute rheumatic fever and certain vagotonic persons. Amer. Heart J. 29:378, 1945.

Robinson, S. J.: Incidence of rheumatic fever in San Francisco children. J. Pediat. 49:272, 1956.

Rosenfeld, A. G.: Children with rheumatic fever in Minnesota. Amer. J. Public Health 48:1596, 1958.

Ross, J., Jr.; Braunwald, E.; and Morrow, A. G.: Clinical hemodynamic observations in pure mitral insufficiency. Amer. J. Cardiol. 2:11, 1958.

Ross, R. S. and Criley, J. M.: Cineangiocardiographic studies of the origin of cardio-vascular physical signs. Circulation 30:255, 1964.

Roth, I. R.; Ling, C.; and Whittemore, A.: Heart disease in children. A rheumatic group. I. Certain aspects of the age at onset and of recurrences in 488 cases of juvenile rheumatism ushered in by major clinical manifestations. Amer. Heart J. 13:36, 1937.

Roy, S. B. and Massell, B. F.: Comparison of large and small doses of hormones in the treatment of acute rheumatic carditis. Circulation 14:44, 1956.

RuDuskey, B. M.: Heart murmurs in youths of military age. J.A.M.A. 185:1004, 1963.

Sabiston, D. C., Jr.; and Follis, R. H., Jr.: Lesions in auricular appendages removed at operations for mitral stenosis of presumed rheumatic origin. Bull. Johns Hopkins Hosp. 91:178, 1952.

Sachs, L.; Feinstein, A. R.; and Taranta, A.: A controlled psychologic study of Sydenham's chorea. J. Pediat. 61:714, 1962.

Saslaw, M. S. and Schwartzman, M. N.: Case registry for rheumatic fever in greater Miami, Florida. Public Health Rep. 77:17, 1962.

Saslaw, M. S. and Streitfield, M. M.: Group A beta hemolytic streptococci and rheu-mátic fever in Miami, Florida: I. Bacteriologic observations from October, 1954 through May, 1955. Dis. Chest 35:175, 1959.

Schlesinger, B.: Subacute infective endocarditis in childhood. Brit. J. Child. Dis 25:33, 1928.

Schlesinger, B.: The relationship of throat infection to acute rheumatism in child-hood. Arch. Dis. Child. 5:411, 1930.

Schmidt, W. C.: Type-specific antibody formation in man following injection of streptococcal M protein. J. Infect. Dis. 106:250, 1960.

Schwab, J. H. and Cromartie, W. J.: Studies on a toxic cellular component of group A streptococci. J. Bact. 74:673, 1957.

Schwartz, S. P. and Schwedel, J. B.: Digital studies on children with heart disease. II. The effects of digitalis on the sinus rate of children with rheumatic fever and chronic valvular heart disease. Amer. J. Dis. Child. 39:298, 1930.

Schwartzman, J.; Zantz, J. B.; and Labow, H.: Chorea-minor: Preliminary report on 6 patients treated with combined A.C.T.H. and cortisone. J. Pediat. 43:278, 1953.

Schwedel, J. B.: Diagnostic value of roentgenography and fluoroscopy in the diag-nosis of rheumatic heart disease. Amer. J. Med. 2:517, 1947.

Segal, J. P.; Harvey, W. P.; and Corrado, M. A.: The Austin Flint murmur: Its dif-ferentiation from the murmur of rheumatic mitral stenosis. Circulation 18:1025, 1958.

Shapiro, M. J.: Differential diagnosis of rheumatic and non-rheumatic leg-pains. Mod. Conc. Cardiov. Dis. 24:295, 1955.

Sharp, J. T.; Hijmans, W.; and Dieves, L.: Examination of the L forms of group A streptococci for the group-specific polysaccharide and M protein. J. Exp. Med. 105:153, 1957.

Sherwood, R. W.; Groubeck, C.; and Denny, F. W., Jr.: Reactions from multiple injections of benzathine penicillin G. J.A.M.A. 165:667, 1957.

Shultz, I.; Gundelfinger, B.; Rosenbaum, M.; Woolridge, R.; and DeBerry, P.: Com-parison of clinical manifestations of respiratory illnesses due to Asian strain influenza, adenovirus and unknown causes. J. Lab. Clin. Med. 55:497, 1960.

Siegel, A. C.; Johnson, E. E.; and Stollerman, G. H.: Controlled studies of strep-tococcal pharyngitis in a pediatric population. I. Factors related to the attack rate of rheumatic fever. New Eng. J. Med. 265:559, 1961.

Simon, H. J. and Sakai, W.: Staphylococcal antagonism to penicillin-G therapy of hemolytic streptococcal pharyngeal infection: Effect of oxacillin. Pediatrics 31:463, 1963.

Smolens, J. and Warner, H. F.: Immunogenic and chemical properties of fractions prepared from ten types of group A streptococci. J. Immun. 68:185, 1952.

Sokoloff, L.: The pathogenesis of rheumatic fever. *In*: Inflammation and Diseases of Connective Tissue, page 135. Ed. Mills, L. C. and Moyer, J. H. W. B. Saunders Co., Philadelphia, 1961.

Spector, W. G. and Willoughby, D. A.: Anti-inflammatory effects of salicylate in the rate. *In*: Salicylates, An International Symposium, page 141. Ed. Dixon, A. St. J., Martin, B. K., Wood, P. H. N. and Smith, M. J. H. Little, Brown and Co., Boston, 1963.

Stamler, J.: Cardiovascular diseases in the United States. Amer. J. Cardiol. *10*:319, 1962.

Stern, A. M.; Sigmann, J. M.; Sloan, H. E.; Strang, R. H.; and Ertel, P. Y.: Relief of severe rheumatic mitral insufficiency in young individuals. Circulation *30*: (Suppl. 3) 167, 1964 (Abs.).

Stetson, C. A., Jr.: The relation of antibody response to rheumatic fever. *In*: Streptococcal Infections, page 208. Columbia University Press, New York, 1954.

Stevenson, A. C. and Cheeseman, E. A.: Heredity and rheumatic fever: A study of 462 families ascertained by an affected child and 51 families ascertained by an affected mother. Ann. Eugen. Lond. *17*:177, 1953.

Stevenson, A. C. and Cheeseman, E. A.: Heredity and rheumatic fever: Some later information about data collected in 1950-51. Ann. Hum. Genet. *21*:139, 1956.

Still, G. F.: Common Disorders and Diseases of Childhood. 3rd ed. Oxford University Press, London, 1918, p. 495.

Stillerman, M. and Bernstein, S. H.: Streptococcal pharyngitis. Amer. J. Dis. Child. *101*:476, 1961.

Stillerman, M. and Bernstein, S. H.: Streptococcal pharyngitis therapy. Amer. J. Dis. Child. *107*:35, 1964.

Stokes, J., III, and Dawber, T. R.: Rheumatic heart disease in the Framingham study. New Eng. J. Med. *255*:1228, 1956.

Stollerman, G. H.: The management and control of rheumatic fever. Acta Rheum. No. 1, North Amer. Series, 1960.

Stollerman, G. H.: Factors determining the attack rate of rheumatic fever. J.A.M.A. *177*:823, 1961.

Stollerman, G. H.: Prognosis and treatment of acute rheumatic fever: The possible effect of treatment on subsequent cardiac disease. Progr. Cardiov. Dis. *3*:193, 1960.

Stollerman, G. H. and Bernheimer, A. W.: Inhibition of streptolysin S by the serum of patients with rheumatic fever and acute streptococcal pharyngitis. J. Clin. Invest. *29*:1147, 1950.

Stollerman, G. H.; Glick, S.; Patel, D. J.; Hirshfeld, I.; and Rusoff, J. H.: Determination of C-reactive protein in serum as a guide to the treatment and management of rheumatic fever. Amer. J. Med. *15*:645, 1953.

Stollerman, G. H.; Lewis, A. J.; Shultz, I.; and Taranta, A.: Relationship of immune response to group A streptococci to the course of acute, chronic and recurrent rheumatic fever. Amer. J. Med. *20*:163, 1956.

Stollerman, G. H. and Rusoff, J. H.: Prophylaxis against group A streptococcal infections in rheumatic fever patients; use of new repository penicillin preparation. J.A.M.A. *150*:1571, 1952.

Stowell, D. D. and Button, W. H., Jr.: Observations on the prophylactic use of sulfonilamide on rheumatic patients with report of one death. J.A.M.A. *117*:2164, 1941.

Streamer, C. W.; Williams, P. M.; Wang, W. L. L.; Johnson, R. S.; McGuire, C. D.; Abelow, I. J.; and Glaser, R. J.: Identification of group A streptococci. Amer. J. Dis. Child. *104*:157, 1962.

Stroud, W. D. and Twaddle, P. H.: Fifteen years' observation of children with rheumatic heart disease. J.A.M.A. *114*:629, 1950.

Sutton, L. P. and Dodge, K. G.: The relationship of Sydenham's chorea to other rheumatic manifestations. Amer. J. Med. Sci. *195*:656, 1938.

Sutton, L. P. and Wyckoff, J.: Digitalis. Its value in the treatment of children with rheumatic heart disease. Amer. J. Dis. Child. *41*:80, 1931.

Swift, H. F.; Hitchcock, C. H.; Derick, C. L.; and McEwen, C.: Intravenous vaccination with streptococci in rheumatic fever. Amer. J. Med. Sci. *181*:1, 1931.

Swift, H. F.; Moen, J. K.; and Hirst, G. K.: The action of sulfanilamide in rheumatic fever. J.A.M.A. *110*:426, 1938.

Taran, L. M.: Rheumatic fever and its relation to dental disease. New York J. Dentistry *14*:107, 1944.

Taran, L. M.; Gulotta, G. A.; Chand, D.; and Angelos, P. H.: Effect of cortisone and ACTH on protracted rheumatic carditis in children. Bull. St. Francis Hosp. (Roslyn) *11*:1, 1954.

Taran, L. M. and Jacobs, M. H.: Salicylate therapy in rheumatic fever in children. J. Pediat. *27*:59, 1945.

Taran, L. M. and Szilaggi, N.: The effect of cardiac rate upon the duration of electrical systole, sinus bradycardia, regular sinus rhythm and sinus tachycardia. Bull. St. Francis Hosp. (Roslyn) *9*:15, 1952.

Taranta, A.: Relation of isolated recurrences of Sydenham's chorea to preceding streptococcal infections. New Eng. J. Med. *260*:1204, 1959.

Taranta, A.: Occurrence of rheumatic-like subcutaneous nodules without evidence of joint or heart disease: Report of a case. New Eng. J. Med. *266*:19, 1962.

Taranta, A.; Kleinberg, E.; Feinstein, A. R.; Wood, H. F.; Tursky, E.; and Simpson, R.: Rheumatic fever in children and adolescents. V. Relation of the rheumatic fever recurrence rate per streptococcal infection to pre-existing clinical features of the patients. Ann. Intern. Med. *60*:(Suppl. 5) 58, 1964.

Taranta, A.; Spagnuolo, M.; and Feinstein, A. R.: "Chronic" rheumatic fever. Ann. Intern. Med. *56*:367, 1962.

Taranta, A. and Stollerman, G. H.: The relationship of Sydenham's chorea to infection with group A streptococci. Amer. J. Med. *20*:170, 1956.

Taranta, A.; Torosdag, S.; Metrakos, J. D.; Jegier, W.; and Uchida, I.: Rheumatic fever in monozygotic and dizygotic twins. Circulation *20*:778, 1959.

Taussig, H. B. and Goldenberg, M.: Roentgenologic studies of size of heart in childhood: 3 different types of teleroentgenographic changes which occur in acute rheumatic fever. Amer. Heart J. *21*:440, 1941.

Tedeschi, C. G.; Wagner, B. M.; and Pani, K. C.: Studies in rheumatic fever. I. The clinical significance of the Aschoff body based on morphologic observations. A.M.A. Arch. Path. *60*:408, 1955.

Thomas, C. B. and France, R.: A preliminary report of the prophylactic use of sulfonamide in patients susceptible to rheumatic fever. Bull. Johns Hopkins Hosp. *64*:67, 1939.

Thomas, L.; Denny, F. W., Jr.; and Floyd, J.: Studies on the generalized Shwartzman reaction. III. Lesions of the myocardium and coronary arteries accompanying the reaction in rabbits prepared by infection with group A streptococci. J. Exp. Med. *97*:751, 1953.

Thomson, S. and Innes, J.: Haemolytic streptococci in the cardiac lesions of acute rheumatism. Brit. Med. J. *2*:733, 1940.

Thorn, G. W.; Jenkins, D.; Laidlaw, J. C.; Goetz, F. C.; Dingman, J. F.; Arons, W. L.; Streeten, D. H. P.; and McCracken, B. H.: Pharmacologic aspects of adrenocortical steroids and ACTH in man. New Eng. J. Med. *248*:232, 1953.

Tillett, W. S. and Francis, T., Jr.: Serological reactions in pneumonia with a nonprotein somatic fraction of pneumococcus. J. Exp. Med. *52*:561, 1930.

Tillett, W. S. and Garner, R. L.: The fibrinolytic activity of hemolytic streptococci. J. Exp. Med. *58*:485, 1933.

Tillett, W. S.; Sherry, S.; and Christensen, L. R.: Streptococcal desoxyribonuclease; significance in lysis of purulent exudates and production by strains of hemolytic streptococci. Proc. Soc. Exp. Biol. Med. *68*:184, 1948.

Todd, E. W.: Antigenic streptococcal hemolysin. J. Exp. Med. *55*:267, 1932.

Todd, E. W.; Coburn, A. F.; and Hill, A. B.: Antistreptolysin S titers in rheumatic fever. Lancet *2*:1213, 1939.

Trousseau, A.: Clinique Médicale de l'Hôtel-Dieu de Paris. 2nd ed. J-B Bailliere et fils, Paris, 1865, vol. 1, p. 106.

Tumulty, P. A.: Antibiotic therapy of bacterial endocarditis. Amer. Heart J. *64*:117, 1962.

Uhr, J. W.: The Streptococcus, Rheumatic Fever and Glomerulonephritis. The Williams and Wilkins Co., Baltimore, 1964.

U. K. and U. S. Joint Report: The treatment of acute rheumatic fever in children: Cooperative clinical trial of ACTH, cortisone and aspirin. Circulation *11*:343 1955.

U. K. and U. S. Joint Report: The evolution of rheumatic heart disease in children: Five year report of a cooperative clinical trial of ACTH, cortisone and aspirin. Circulation *22*:503, 1960.

U. S. Department of Health, Education and Welfare. Public Health Service: A manual for a rheumatic fever registry, 1961.

U. S. Department of Health, Education and Welfare. Public Health Service Publication no. 1083. Cardiovascular disease: 1960 Data on national and state mortality experience. U. S. Government Printing Office, Washington, D.C., 1964.

Usher, S. J. and Jasper, H.: The etiology of Sydenham's chorea: Electroencephalographic studies. Canad. Med. Ass. J. *44*:365, 1941.

Uzsoy, N. K.: The coexistence of rheumatic heart disease and sickle cell anemia. Amer. J. Med. Sci. *246*:462, 1963.

Vazquez, J. J. and Dixon, F. J.: Immunohistochemical analysis of lesions associated with "fibrinoid change." A.M.A. Arch. Path. *66*:504, 1958.

VonGlahn, W. C.: The pathology of rheumatism. Amer. J. Med. *2*:76, 1947.

Wagner, B. M.: Studies in rheumatic fever. III. Histochemical reactivity of the Aschoff body. Ann. N. Y. Acad. Sci. *86*:992, 1960.

Wagner, V. and Rejholec, V.: Agglutinins and incomplete antibodies after a single antigenic inoculation in normal and rheumatic individuals. Ann. Rheum. Dis. *14*:243, 1955.

Wallace, H. L. and Smith, A. B.: The effect of early tonsillectomy on the incidence of acute rheumatism. Edinburgh M. J. *43*:452, 1936.

Wallgren, A.: Studies on erythema annulare rheumaticum. Acta paediat. *17*:447, 1935.

Wannamaker, L. W.: The differentiation of three distinct desoxyribonucleases of group A streptococci. J. Exp. Med. *107*:797, 1958.

Wannamaker, L. W.: Characterization of a fourth desoxyribonuclease of group A streptococci. Fed. Proc. *21*:231, 1962 (Abst.).

Wannamaker, L. W.: Streptococcal desoxyribonucleases. *In*: The Streptococcus, Rheumatic Fever and Glomerulonephritis, page 140. Ed. Uhr, J. W. The Williams and Wilkins Co., Baltimore, 1964.

Wannamaker, L. W. and Ayoub, E. M.: Antibody titers in acute rheumatic fever. Circulation *21*:598, 1960.

Wannamaker, L. W.; Denny, F. W.; Perry, W. D.; Rammelkamp, C. H., Jr.; Eckhardt, G. C.; Houser, H. B.; and Hahn, E. O.: The effect of penicillin prophylaxis on streptococcal disease rate and the carrier state. New Eng. J. Med. *249*:1, 1953.

Wannamaker, L. W.; Rammelkamp, C. H., Jr.; Denny, F. W.; Brink, W. R.; Houser, H. B.; Hahn, E. O.; and Dingle, J. H.: Prophylaxis of acute rheumatic fever by treatment of the preceding streptococcal infection with various amounts of depot penicillin. Amer. J. Med. *10*:673, 1951.

Warfield, M. A.; Page, R. H.; Zuelzer, W. W.; and Stulberg, C. S.: Immunofluorescence in diagnostic bacteriology. II. Identification of group A streptococci in throat smears. Amer. J. Dis. Child. *101*:160, 1961.

Watkinson, G.: Massive salicylate therapy in rheumatic fever. Ann. Rheum. Dis. *8*:120, 1949.

Watson, R. F.; Hirst, G. K.; and Lancefield, R. C.: Bacteriological studies of cardiac tissues obtained at autopsy from eleven patients dying with rheumatic fever. Arthritis Rheum. *4*:74, 1961.

Watson, R. F.; Rothbard, S.; and Swift, H. F.: The use of penicillin in rheumatic fever. J.A.M.A. *126*:274, 1944.

Watson, R. F.; Rothbard, S.; and Swift, H. F.: Type-specific protection and immunity following intranasal inoculation of monkeys with group A hemolytic streptococci. J. Exp. Med. *84*:127, 1946.

Wedum, B. G. and McGuire, J. W.: Origin of the Aschoff body. Ann. Rheum. Dis. *22*:127, 1963.

Wells, B.: The assessment of mitral stenosis by phonocardiography. Brit. Heart J. *16*:261, 1954.

White, P. D.: Changes in relative prevalence of various types of heart disease in New England. Contrast between 1925 and 1950. J.A.M.A. *152*:303, 1953.

Wilson, M. G.: Rheumatic Fever; Studies of the Epidemiology, Manifestations, Diagnosis and Treatment of the Disease during the First Three Decades. The Commonwealth Fund, New York; London-Humphrey Milford, Oxford University Press, 1940.

Wilson, M. G.: Present status of hormone therapy in rheumatic fever with special reference to short-term treatment in active carditis. Advances Pediat. *11*:243, 1960.

Wilson, M. G.: Advances in Rheumatic Fever, 1940-1961. Harper and Row, New York, 1962.

Wilson, M. G.; Helper, H. N.; Lubschez, R.; Hain, K.; and Epstein, N.: Effect of short-term administration of corticotropin in active rheumatic carditis. A.M.A. Amer. J. Dis. Child. *86*:131, 1953.

Wilson, M. G. and Lim, W. N.: Natural course of active rheumatic carditis and evaluation of hormone therapy. J.A.M.A. *160*:1457, 1956.

Wilson, M. G. and Lim, W. N.: Short-term hormone therapy: Its effect in active rheumatic carditis of varying duration. New Eng. J. Med. *260*:802, 1959.

Wilson, M. G. and Lubschez, R.: Recurrence rates in rheumatic fever. The evaluation of etiologic concepts and consequent preventive therapy. J.A.M.A. *126*:477, 1944.

Wilson, M. G. and Schweitzer, M.: Pattern of hereditary susceptibility in rheumatic fever. Circulation *10*:699, 1954.

Wilson, M. G.; Schweitzer, M. D.; and Lubschez, R.: The familial epidemiology of rheumatic fever: Genetic and epidemiologic studies; genetic studies. J. Pediat. *22*:468, 581, 1943.

Wilson, M. G. and Swift, H. F.: Intravenous vaccination with hemolytic streptococci: Its influence on the incidence of recurrences of rheumatic fever in children. Amer. J. Dis. Child. *42*:42, 1931.

Winkelman, N. W. and Eckel, J. L.: Endarteritis of small cortical vessels in severe infections and toxemias. Arch. Neurol. and Psychiat. *21*:863, 1929.

Wintrobe, M. M.: Clinical Hematology. 4th ed. Lea and Febiger, Philadelphia, 1956, p. 320.

Wittler, R. G.; Tuckett, J. D.; Muccione, V. J.; Gangarosa, E. J.; and O'Connell, R. C.: Transition forms and L forms from the blood of rheumatic fever patients. International (8) Congress of Microbiology, Abstracts, p. 125, 1962.

Wolfe, C. K.; Hayaski, J. A.; Walsh, G.; and Barkulis, S. S.: Type-specific antibody response in man to injections of cell walls and M protein from group A, type 4 streptococci. J. Lab. Clin. Med. *61*:459, 1963.

Wood, H. F.; Feinstein, A. R.; Taranta, A.; Epstein, J. A.; and Simpson, R.: Rheumatic fever in children and adolescents. III. Comparative effectiveness of three prophylaxis regimens in preventing streptococcal infections and rheumatic recurrences. Ann. Intern. Med. *60*:(Suppl. 5) 31, 1964.

Wood, H. F. and McCarty, M.: Laboratory aids in the diagnosis of rheumatic fever and in evaluation of disease activity. Amer. J. Med. *17*:768, 1954.

Wood, H. F.; McCarty, M.; and Slater, R. J.: The occurrence during acute infections of a protein not normally present in the blood: V. Physical-chemical properties of the C-reactive protein crystallized by a modified technique. J. Exp. Med. *100*:71, 1954.

Woodward, T. E.; McCrumb, F. R., Jr.; Carey, T. N.; and Togo, Y.: Viral and rickettsial causes of cardiac disease, including the Coxsackie virus etiology of pericarditis and myocarditis. Ann. Intern. Med. *53*:1130, 1960.

Yearbook of Pediatrics. Gellis, S. S. ed. 1959-1960 series, p. 289. Year Book Medical Publishers, Chicago.

Yuan, S-H.; Doyle, E. F.; Pisacano, J. C.; and Reed, G. E.: Severe rheumatic mitral insufficiency in childhood amenable to surgery. Pediatrics *33*:571, 1964.

Zabriskie, J. B.: The role of temperate bacteriophage in the production of erythrogenic toxin by group A streptococci. J. Exp. Med. *119*:761, 1964.

Zabriskie, J. B.; Freimer, E. H.; and Seegal, B.: An immunological relationship between streptococcal membranes and human heart tissue. Fed. Proc. 23:342, 1964 (Abst.).

Ziegra, S. R. and Kuttner, A. G.: Reappearance of abnormal laboratory findings in rheumatic patients following withdrawal of ACTH or cortisone (with special reference to the C-reactive protein). Amer. J. Med. Sci. 222:(new series) 516, 1951.

Zimmerman, R. A.; Siegel, A. C.; and Steele, C. P.: An epidemiological investigation of a streptococcal and rheumatic fever epidemic in Dickenson, North Dakota. Pediatrics 30:712, 1962.

Index